HEALTH COMMUNICATION, *16*(1), 1–5

"Collective Amnesia:" The Absence of Religious Faith and Spirituality in Health Communication Research and Practice

Roxanne Parrott

Department of Communication Arts & Sciences
The Pennsylvania State University

Health communication has focused largely on the translation of expert discourse into medical and public health messages for dissemination to lay audiences as a strategy to influence health beliefs and behaviors. Recognition that many health beliefs and behaviors are formed, maintained, and reinforced in less formal settings and not strategically designed to influence has increased health communication research associated with lay discourse about health and health care. This is especially true among health communicators who herald communication as their primary field of expertise (e.g., Beach, 2002; Condit, Parrott, & Harris, 2002; Parrott, Silk, & Condit, 2003). In conjunction with such work is recognition that lay theories about health and health care, which are often unspoken, impede efforts to understand expert discourse (Rowan, 2000). A primary premise of this special issue is that religious faith and spirituality comprise an integral component of lay discourse and lay theories associated with health. Individual predisposition to think, feel, or act based on belief in a spiritual power greater than humans affecting the course of nature and the role of humans within that realm has far-reaching health effects. Knowledge about lay discourse associated with religious faith and spirituality, therefore, is likely to reveal insights about lay theories associated with health, which may be used to facilitate health education, promotion, and counseling efforts across disciplinary boundaries associated with health communication.

Literally hundreds of published empirical studies have explored relations between religion and physical health. One review in the early 1990s found more than 300 studies in a range of fields that included epidemiology, gerontology, and the

Requests for reprints should be sent to Roxanne Parrott, The Pennsylvania State University, Department of Communication Arts & Sciences, University Park, PA 16802. E-mail: rlp18@psu.edu behavioral sciences (Levin & Vanderpool, 1991). Another review of published research in mental health nursing journals for the years 1991 through 1995 found that 10% of the articles included a measure of religion or spirituality—an eightfold increase over a previous review (Weaver, Flannelly, Flannelly, Koenig, & Larson, 1998). In 2002, the *Annals of Behavioral Medicine* published a special issue devoted to the topic of "Spirituality, Religiousness, and Health: From Research to Clinical Practice" (Mills, 2002). Despite these widespread collections of evidence regarding relations between religious faith and health, literature regarding the study of religious faith and spirituality in health communication is sparse to none. Within the field of communication more broadly, publications relating to religious faith are also few but include a program of research about communication and prayer (Baesler, 1999), reviews highlighting religion's role in contributing to successful aging for older adults (Nussbaum, Pecchioni, Robinson, & Thompson, 2000), and work relating religious faith to identity formation (Hecht, Jackson, & Ribeau, 2003). Thus, the articles included in this collection begin to fill a void and, at the same time, illustrate a role health communication fulfills within the behavioral sciences, emphasizing how everyday people make sense of health conditions in their everyday living.

Following this introduction, Egbert, Mickley, and Coeling (this issue) provide an integrated synthesis of the ways and means that religious faith and spirituality have been assessed, primarily through use of quantitative measures. Their review strategically sets the stage for understanding the evolution of research designed to operationalize religious faith and spirituality, as well as how and where health communication might be situated in this complex topic. The next two articles utilize instruments discussed in the Egbert et al. review. Parrott, Silk, Krieger, Harris, and Condit (this issue) propose a model of media exposure and effects associated with intrinsic and extrinsic religiosity. They use two of the most widely tested instruments associated with religious faith to examine its role on media use and behavioral health outcomes associated with human genetics. Soweid, Khawaja, and Salem (this issue) relate religious identity to the smoking behavior of University of Beirut college students and discuss the role of this knowledge in guiding audience segmentation, as well as its potential for social norming campaigns that might refer to expectations associated with religious faith and smoking behavior.

The remaining articles in this issue utilize qualitative methods to begin to address the absence of specific understanding regarding religious faith and health communication, answering the challenge to health communicators to enrich the field through greater use of such methodological approaches to inquiry (du Pre, 2002; Query & Wright, 2003). Robinson and Nussbaum (this issue) consider the frequency with which references to religious faith and practices occur during medical interaction, offering discussion about the value of listening for such references to guide clinical insights. Keeley (this issue) looks at discourse during final conversations and finds that references to religious faith and spirituality are common, functioning to validate the human experience and comfort survivors. Harris, Parrott, and Dorgan's (this issue) examination of how lay audiences talk about the role of God or a "Higher Power" in genes and health fills in some of the gaps associated with lay theories that guide decision making in this context. Anderson's (this issue) research regarding parish nurse programs and the experiences of nurse participants may enrich health communication scholars' understanding of social support, especially esteem support. Insights about health care delivery and health promotion of health in faith-based settings are also provided.

All contributors to this special issue confront the ethical parameters associated with including religious faith and spirituality in health communication research, for there are many related concerns. Perhaps the fallow field relates in part to statements such as the following:

> While many researchers continue to produce empirical evidence for salutary religious effects, the emergence of this field of inquiry has suffered from a sort of collective amnesia on the part of social scientists, epidemiologists, and biomedical professionals whose tacit professional knowledge tends to downplay the role of religious belief and involvement as salient influences upon health. As a result, only in recent years have linkages between religion and health begun to be exploited for purposes of health promotion and disease prevention. (Levin & Vanderpool, 1991, p. 42)

The authors then cite a brochure developed by the Department of Health and Human Services related to the use of churches as a site to promote blood pressure control.

Many health communicators—myself included—will likely react to the notion of "exploiting" religious faith. The implication is that because individuals gather at a site of worship, it affords a situation in which blood pressure control screenings and education will be passively received and compliance more likely. An alternative way of viewing the situation is to consider that an obligation to make sense of churchgoers' habits has been recognized, and outreach to a church setting makes a program accessible to an audience that might otherwise not have access. Efforts to derive knowledge about the role of religious faith to guide strategic health communication necessarily requires concerned and concerted ethical analysis, however, with guidelines toward that purpose provided by each contributor. Health communicators also should not add to the "collective amnesia" alluded to earlier, as religious faith and spirituality often direct the thoughts, feelings, and actions of many of us, giving life and—as Keeley affirms—death meaning. The contributors to this special issue acknowledge this reality, suggesting the theoretical and practical outcomes of their work, and advancing ideas for future research.

In many ways, the contributions to this special issue distinguish health communication derived from communication theory and practice from other fields with some overlap in the interdisciplinary pursuit of communicating about health.

Health communicators who emphasize communication theory and practice often acknowledge barriers to disclosure in their research and teaching. Among the lessons summarized from such work is the fact that societal taboos impact communication about health, and, therefore, health beliefs and behaviors (Petronio, 2000). These often unwritten rules prescribe what we talk about and with whom, as well as how and when. The effects of taboos for health have been well-illustrated with regard to sex, death and dying, alcohol consumption, drug use, and a myriad of lifestyle issues. Absent from these collections of knowledge about taboos, however, is reference to religious faith and spirituality, a situation that begins to change with this collection.

This special issue closes with a note from Dr. Michael Long, the Senior Minister in my own church home for nearly a decade and the pastor who performed my daughter's wedding, someone with whom I have served locally on Church and Society committees and abroad in Mexico on mission trips. Thus, I acknowledge my own religious faith and spirituality, which parallels the experience of one of the reviewers who, in reading some of the submitted work that was revised and is included in the contents of this special issue said, "Isn't it just so obvious?" As the flagship academic publication outlet for health communication research, one role of this journal is to bring to the foreground assumptions long held but too often invisible in efforts to explain the multifaceted decision-making processes associated with individual well-being. Discourse associated with religious faith and spirituality illustrates this premise.

ACKNOWLEDGMENTS

The reviewers for this special issue significantly contributed to the quality and contents of this issue, and I am most grateful for their expertise. They include individuals cited in the introduction whose own published research has contributed to awareness that religious faith and spirituality constitute vital topics too long ignored in health communication, as well as individuals who have emphasized the need for broader methodological approaches to building knowledge in health communication. The reviewers were Walid Afifi, Michael Hecht, and Jon Nussbaum, Department of Communication Arts & Sciences, The Pennsylvania State University, University Park, PA; E. James Baesler, Communication and Theatre Arts, Old Dominion University, Norfolk, VA; Athena duPre, Department of Communication Arts, University of West Florida, Pensacola, FL; Mary Beth Oliver, Department of Film/Video and Media Studies, The Pennsylvania State University, University Park, PA; and Jim Query, School of Communication, University of Houston, Houston, TX.

REFERENCES

Baesler, E. J. (1999). A model of interpersonal Christian prayer. *Journal of Communication and Religion, 22,* 40–64.

Beach, W. A. (2002). Between dad and son: Initiating, delivering, and assimilating bad cancer news. *Health Communication, 14,* 271–298.

Condit, C. M., Parrott, R., & Harris, T. M. (2002). Lay understandings of the relationship between race and genetics: Development of a collectivized knowledge through shared discourse. *Public Understanding of Science, 11,* 373–387.

du Pre, A. (2002). Accomplishing the impossible: Talking about body and soul and mind during a medical visit. *Health Communication, 14,* 1–22.

Hecht, M. L., Jackson, R. L., & Ribeau, S. (2003). *African American communication: Exploring identity and culture* (2nd ed.). Mahwah, NJ: Lawrence Erlbaum and Associates, Inc.

Levin, J. S., & Vanderpool, H. Y. (1991). Religious factors in physical health and the prevention of illness. *Prevention in Human Services, 9*(2), 41–64.

Mills, P. J. (2002). Spirituality, religiousness, and health: From research to clinical practice. *Annals of Behavioral Medicine, 24,* 1–2.

Nussbaum, J. F., Pecchioni, L. L., Robinson, J. D., & Thompson, T. L. (2000). *Communication and aging.* Mahwah, NJ: Lawrence Erlbaum Associates, Inc.

Parrott, R., Silk, K., & Condit, C. (2003). Diversity in lay perceptions of the sources of human traits: Genes, environments, and personal behaviors. *Social Science & Medicine, 56,* 1099–1109.

Petronio, S. (2000). *Balancing the secrets of private disclosures.* Mahwah, NJ: Lawrence Erlbaum Associates, Inc.

Query, J. L., & Wright, K. B. (2003). Assessing communication competence in an online study: Toward informing subsequent interventions among older adults with cancer, their lay caregivers, and peers. *Health Communication, 15,* 205–219.

Rowan, K. E. (2000). Explaining illness through the mass media: The problem-solving perspective. In B. B. Whaley (Ed.), *Explaining illness: Research, theory, and strategies* (pp. 69–100). Mahwah, NJ: Lawrence Erlbaum Associates, Inc.

Weaver, A. J., Flannelly, L. T., Flannelly, K. J., Koenig, H. G., & Larson, D. B. (1998). An analysis of research on religious and spiritual variables in three major mental health nursing journals. *Issues in Mental Health Nursing, 19,* 263–276.

HEALTH COMMUNICATION, *16*(1), 7–27

A Review and Application of Social Scientific Measures of Religiosity and Spirituality: Assessing a Missing Component in Health Communication Research

Nichole Egbert
School of Communication Studies
Kent State University

Jacqueline Mickley
Hospice and Supportive Care
Visiting Nurse Service

Harriet Coeling
College of Nursing
Kent State University

Social and behavioral scientists in fields such as psychology, sociology, anthropology, nursing, and medicine have been investigating the relation between religious or spiritual variables and health outcomes for several decades. This article reviews a sample of the major empirical instruments used in this research, including extrinsic and intrinsic religiosity, spiritual well-being, and religious coping. The review encompasses suggestions for application of these scales to health communication theory and research associated with identity, self-efficacy, social support, and media use. Cautionary advice regarding ethical issues together with guidelines for use is advanced.

In their poll of 60 countries ($N = 50,000$), the Gallup International Millennium Survey reported that 87% of respondents consider themselves to be members of

Requests for reprints should be sent to Nichole Egbert, School of Communication Studies, P.O. Box 5190, Kent State University, Kent, OH 44242. E-mail: negbert@kent.edu some religion. In North America specifically, 62% believe that there is a personal God, 24% believe that there is some sort of spirit or life force, and 83% give God high importance in their lives (Carballo, n. d.). Despite its prevalence, up until the early 1980s, many clinicians and researchers avoided the study of religiosity and spirituality (RS), as perhaps the subject seemed too ethereal, unscientific, or controversial (Larimore, Parker, & Crowther, 2002; Levin, 1994; Pargament & Park, 1995). That picture has changed as scholars realize the multifarious and extensive influence that religion and spirituality can have on individuals' health beliefs and practices (T. W. Smith, 2001; Zinnbauer, Pargament, & Scott, 1999). Although there are skeptics (i.e., Sloan & Bagiella, 2002), most health researchers remain open-minded and optimistic about the possibility of an association between religion and spirituality and health outcomes (Levin, 1994; Thoreson & Harris, 2002).

The purpose of this review is not to convince the reader of the verity of the faith–health connection. The goal is to introduce some of the empirical instruments that are available, assess their communication content, comment on their utility for communication research, and review some relevant ethical considerations. As the majority of published measures assess RS variables using quantitative self-report instruments, this review emphasizes quantitative approaches over qualitative, although both strategies enhance understanding of religion and health. Before relevant measures can be reviewed, definitions of religiousness and spirituality are addressed.

DEFINING RELIGIOUSNESS AND SPIRITUALITY

Operational definitions of spirituality and religiousness have been vague and contradictory in past research (Koenig, McCullough, & Larson 2001), and thus there has been interest in clarifying the concepts. Spirituality is commonly viewed as individual experiences relating to God or a higher power, as well as existential aspirations of finding meaning and purpose in life (Kirkwood, 1994; Moberg, 2002; Thoresen, Harris, & Oman, 2001). Religiousness is commonly viewed as society-based beliefs and practices relating to God or a higher power commonly associated with a church or organized group (Thoresen et al., 2001; Zinnbauer et al., 1999). Many researchers argue that both spirituality and religiousness are multidimensional constructs with unique characteristics that have overlapping dimensions (Paloutzian & Kirkpatrick, 1995; Thoreson & Harris, 2002). Larson, Swyers, and McCullough (1998) concluded that both spirituality and religiousness involve the cognitions, emotions, and behaviors involved with searching for the sacred. In an effort to be as inclusive as possible when dealing with these terms, Thoreson and Harris (2002) recommended using the term *Religious/Spiritual Measures* to denote measurement of these constructs. The abbreviation RS is used in this article to designate religious or spiritual variables and concepts.

GENERAL MEASURES OF RELIGIOUS
BELIEF AND PRACTICE

The following section is a review of some of the most widely used RS instruments, as well as descriptions of RS measures of particular interest to health communication researchers. For the sake of breadth of application, no single health communication theory or orientation will be spotlighted in this review. Throughout the discussion, examples of several theories used by health communication scholars are offered in relation to relevant RS instruments. Although numerous book chapters, handbooks, and journal articles provide information regarding RS measures, readers are referred especially to Hill and Hood (1999), Koenig et al. (2001), and Plante and Sherman (2001). These resources provide excellent summaries, as well as additional information regarding the reliability, validity, and specific items used in measures of RS.

Measures of Intrinsic and Extrinsic Religiosity

Allport and Ross (1967) differentiated between extrinsically and intrinsically motivated individuals by saying that, "the extrinsically motivated person *uses* his religion, whereas the intrinsically motivated *lives* his religion" (p. 434). Allport and Ross argued that the extrinsic orientation is "instrumental and utilitarian" (p. 434), whereas the intrinsically oriented individual brings everything in life to be in concert with religious belief.

Religious orientation scale (ROS). This early and influential instrument contains 20 items; 11 of which measure extrinsic religiosity (i.e., "What religion offers me most is comfort when sorrows and misfortune strike," and "One reason for my being a church member is that such membership helps to establish a person in the community"), and 9 intrinsic religiosity items (i.e., "If I were to join a church group I would prefer to join a Bible study group rather than a social fellowship," and "Quite often I have been keenly aware of the presence of God or the Divine Being"). Allport and Ross's (1967) Intrinsic–Extrinsic scale has prompted a wide range of research, yet has also received criticism for its Christian bias and problems related to social desirability (Burris, 1999b; Kirkpatrick & Hood, 1990). In a meta-analysis of 34 studies, Donahue (1985) concluded that the intrinsic religiousness scale is usable with Christian denominations, but as of 1982 had not shown any significant correlations with any other variables except other measures of religiousness. Extrinsic religiousness often correlates positively with traditionally negative traits such as prejudice, dogmatism, and fear of death (Allport & Ross, 1967; Donahue, 1985). Hunsberger (1996) clarified this claim, arguing that extrinsic religiosity is associated with prejudice only when it takes the form of right-wing authoritarianism. The I–E subscales are further distinguished in that the intrinsic scale typically shows better internal consistency (in the mid-.80s) than the extrinsic scale (mid-.70s). Due to the fact that this scale has evolved through many revisions, it is difficult to locate health studies that used this original formulation of the I–E scale.

The division of the RS variable into intrinsic and extrinsic religiosity represents a slight paradigm shift for social science researchers. Due to this bifurcation, health communication scholars can explore communication behavior as it relates to both individual difference variables and social and community relationships, linking these to health outcomes. For example, some researchers who study social support and health may be interested in the structural aspects of social support networks and communities, which would be best assessed through a measure of extrinsic religiosity. On the other hand, those who are interested in the psychological aspects of supportive relationships, such as the communicative competence of support providers (e.g., Query & Kreps, 1996), perceived availability of social support (e.g., Conn & Peterson, 1989), and the actual messages used in conveying support to a recipient (e.g., Burleson, 1983), may be more interested in the degree to which intrinsic religiousness influences these processes. In the early stages of this research, both aspects should be included to determine which concept provides the most predictive power when investigating social support and health outcomes.

Age universal I–E scale.   As mentioned in the last section, several offshoots of Allport and Ross's (1967) ROS scale have been created. Most notably, a modified version of Allport and Ross's I–E ROS was produced by Gorsuch and Venable (1983) and was termed the *Age Universal* for use with populations in various stages of human development. This instrument includes all 20 items of the original scale, but uses simpler language and is "completely interchangeable with the Allport and Ross scale" (Hill, 1999, p. 121). Reliability for the Age Universal scale has been good for university students and adults (Maltby, 1999; Maltby & Lewis, 1996), but not much data is available for its internal consistency with younger samples. One notable exception is a study by Gorsuch and Venable (1983) that reported alpha coefficients of .75 for external religiosity and .68 for internal religiosity in a sample of 230 fifth- and seventh-grade students. Although the scales have been used in a study examining racial differences in an elderly sample (Nelson, 1989), few studies have used the scale in health research. Another criticism of the scale is that its items are worded in such a way that religiosity is assumed, for example, "I enjoy reading about my religion," or "My whole approach to life is based on my religion." Therefore, this scale would be inappropriate for use with nonreligious samples.

To address this deficiency, Maltby and Lewis (1996) changed the instructions to participants and constructed an amended age universal I–E scale that improved both the scale's reliability and validity. The revised scale changed the response options from the traditional *strongly agree* to *strongly disagree* to *Does the attitude or behaviour described in the statement apply to me?* with response options of *yes, not certain,* and *no* (Maltby & Lewis, 1996, p. 940). The newer version increased response rates and reliability coefficients and provided a clearer factor structure than the original Age Universal I–E scale. Due to its simplicity and compatibility with the original I–E ROS, this revised scale may be useful to health communication researchers studying college student populations.

Intrinsic religious motivation scale (IRMS).   Hoge's (1972) scale is taken in part from Allport and Ross's (1967) ROS. Hoge's measure is attractive to communication researchers because its 10 items focus on motivations behind faith and religion rather than on the frequency of religious behavior (both of which were included in the Allport & Ross, 1967, scale). Sample items include the following: "One should seek God's guidance when making every important decision," and "My religious beliefs are what really lie behind my whole approach to life." The IRMS is also attractive because it is general enough to be applied to various religious groups (Bassett, 1999). Three of the items are negatively worded, and although it can be argued that these three items form an extrinsic religiosity subscale, reverse-scoring them results in a unidimensional intrinsic religiosity subscale with acceptable reliability and construct validity in medical samples (Hoge, 1972; Sherman & Simonton, 2001). In addition, Benson et al. (1980) demonstrated evidence that intrinsic religiousness (assessed through Hoge's, 1972, scale) was a significant positive predictor of nonspontaneous helping (e.g., volunteering, giving to charity, etc.). There are studies in the realm of clinical research, such as the one by Pargament et al. (1992), that included the scale when studying a sample of 569 adults coping with a negative life event such as illness or injury or the death of a close friend or family member.

Motivation has become an important consideration in health communication research (e.g., Lipkus, 2001; Vishwanath, Kahn, Finnegan, Hertog, & Potter, 1993). Learning how to motivate individuals to take a proactive stance on their health or to seek health-related information is an enduring challenge in our field. Religious motivation, especially intrinsic religiousness scales such as Hoge's (1972) instrument, may shed new light on how some populations process information about health risk. RS motivation serves a different communicative function than either emotional or cognitive appeals and could be explored as an additional tool in motivating health promotion activities.

Quest scale.   Apart from intrinsic and extrinsic religiousness, a third motivational factor, one's search for answers to ultimate questions, has been represented in Batson and Schoenrade's (1991a, 1991b) Quest scale. This 12-item instrument measures the "(a) 'readiness to face existential questions without reducing their complexity,' '(b) self-criticism and perceptions of religious doubts as positive,' and (c) 'openness to change'" (Burris, 1999b, p. 148). Examples of items include, "I am constantly questioning my religious beliefs," and "I was not very interested in religion until I began to ask questions about the meaning and purpose of my life." There are several potential psychometric and construct validity problems with Batson and Schoenrade's (1991a) scale, including poor internal consistency (Sherman & Simonton, 2001; Slater, Hall, & Edwards, 2001). An amended version of the Quest scale has also been constructed that is more applicable to both religious and nonreligious samples (Maltby & Day, 1998). Although the Quest scales address a unique dimension of spiritual maturity and could be used with a broad range of samples, so far they have mainly been tested with college students and have not been used in health-related studies (Koenig et al., 2001; Sherman & Simonton, 2001).

In health communication research, much work is being conducted around the idea of uncertainty (e.g., Babrow, Hines, & Kasch, 2000; Brashers et al., 2000). Babrow's (1992) Problematic Integration Theory, in particular, focuses on how people cope with the unknown factors related to illness (Babrow et al., 2000). Scales such as the Quest scales, which highlight one's ability to search for answers and one's comfort with the unknowable, seem particularly appropriate to these lines of investigation. Perhaps future studies will uncover how one's search for meaning in life may be related to one's search for meaning in health and illness.

Duke religion index (DUREL).   A sample of three items from Hoge's (1972) scale were included in the very brief Duke Religion Index (DUREL; Koenig, Meador, & Parkerson, 1997), an instrument designed explicitly for measuring religious variables related to health outcomes (Koenig et al., 2001). Koenig and colleagues have developed this scale with populations including psychiatric (Koenig et al., 1997) and cardiovascular patients (Koenig et al., 1998). When tested in a study of bone marrow transplant and gynecology clinic patients, the three items from Hoge's scale that tap intrinsic religiosity demonstrated acceptable reliability and consistency to the longer IRMS (Sherman et al., 2000). The other two dimensions, organizational religiousness (OR) and nonorganizational religiousness (NOR), involve asking respondents to indicate how often they attend church or religious meetings (OR) and how often they spend time in private religious activities such as prayer or Bible study (NOR). Little is known about the reliability of the instrument in its entirety. The one-item measurement of OR and NOR allows for easy administration, but the brevity limits reliability estimates (Sherman & Simonton, 2001).

The simplicity of the DUREL and its design for use in health samples make it applicable to topics such as gaining compliance in organ donation (e.g., Miller, 2002; Morgan & Miller, 2002). Morgan and Miller focused on the effects of attitudes, knowledge, altruism, and demographic variables on tendencies to communicate about organ donation. Basic measures of RS variables may add insight into issues related to demographics, but also to how religious or nonreligious families communicate about organ donation, helping others, and the importance placed on the physical remains of the body after death.

Attitude toward Christianity scales.   Researchers looking to assess intrinsic religiosity of a Christian sample may want to consider the 12-item Francis and Stubbs (1987) Attitude Toward Christianity Scale, or the shorter, seven-item Short Scale of Attitude Towards Christianity Scale (Adamson, Shevlin, Lloyd, & Lewis, 2000; Maltby & Lewis, 1997). The scale appears to be highly reliable and unidimensional, but has yet to be tested widely in health-related projects. Sample items include "I know that Jesus helps me," and "God means a lot to me."

Santa Clara strength of religious faith (SCSORF).   One of the few instruments not reviewed in the volume edited by Hill and Hood (1999), this scale is found in a report by Lewis, Shevlin, McGuckin, and Navratil (2001) who provided evidence of the measure's acceptable unidimensional factor structure. Items include "My religious faith is extremely important to me," and "I look to my faith as a source of comfort." The scale is appropriate for use across religious denomination or affiliation with the inclusion of words such as "church" and "God," but perhaps not as appropriate for non-Christian samples. Other studies have found the SCSORF to have good convergent validity and high internal reliability (see Sherman & Simonton, 2001, for a review). In some medical samples, such as women receiving gynecologic attention and patients receiving bone marrow transplants, the SCSORF has high correlations with other measures of religion, but only modest correlations with variables such as social support and optimism (Sherman & Simonton, 2001). Further testing of the SCSORF is needed, as little attention has been paid to this measure outside the work of Plante and colleagues (Lewis et al., 2001).

Index of core spiritual experiences (INSPIRIT).   If researchers are looking for a scale that is even broader than these measures of religious faith, yet need an instrument that is conceptually similar to the Intrinsic Religiosity scales of Allport and Ross (1967) or Hoge (1972), the INSPIRIT might be used (Koenig et al., 2001). The INSPIRIT was designed for use with health outcomes research and to "identify experiences that are described in more intense or concrete terms than an amorphous 'belief in God'" (Hinebaugh-Igoe, 1999, p. 361). The two-factor instrument measures one's convictions of God's existence (three items; i.e., "How often have you felt as though you were very close to a powerful spiritual force that seemed to lift you outside yourself?") and one's beliefs and actions related to a closeness with God (four items; i.e., "How strongly religious (or spiritually oriented) do you consider yourself to be?"). The instrument has acceptable reliability and construct validity with internal religiousness, but has suffered some criticism about the checklist format of one item and lack of variability in samples in which it has been tested (Hinebaugh-Igoe, 1999). Health researchers who have used the INSPIRIT include Kass, Friedman, Lesserman, Zuttermeister, and Benson (1991), who tested the scale with medical out-patients, and VandeCreek, Ayres, and Bassham, (1995), who used the scale with a group of individuals living with cancer and their families. Health communication researchers who may be interested in this scale include those studying traumatic events, such as near-death experiences, or communication about end-of-life issues.

Denominational and Culture-Specific Measures of RS

Although some would argue that, for the sake of generalizability, a more inclusive approach is better for assessing RS variables (T. W. Smith, 2001), others stress that religious groups often focus on their uniqueness, and that failing to take differences of faith and practice into account will only result in a less sophisticated understanding of the RS construct (Moberg, 2002; Thoreson & Harris, 2002). Although denominational measures of RS variables are much less established as compared with more "universal" measures often used in health research, researchers should be aware of the existence of instruments that are denominationally or religion-specific. A list of these measures and their sources is available in Koenig et al. (2001), including measures for Jewish, Hindu, Muslim, Buddhist, and Christian (Orthodox and non-Orthodox) samples.

Researchers studying African American populations may desire measures that reflect traditional African American religious values and culture. Several studies have begun to adjust existing instruments or constructed new culture-specific measurement tools. In a study of collectivism, racial pride, and time orientation in urban African American women, Lukwago, Bucholtz, Kreuter, Holt, and Clark (2001) borrowed nine items from existing scales and constructed two more for a religiosity scale (α = .89). Jagers and Smith (1996) constructed a measure of spirituality that reflects an Afrocultural perspective and may relate well to projects with health-related data. This 20-item measure of spirituality (alphas ranging from .84 to .87) includes items such as, "To me, everything has some amount of spiritual quality," and "Though I may go to the doctor when I am ill, I also pray," (p. 433). Finally, in a study of African American Catholic men, religiosity was measured in three categories (each with multiple indicators): impact of parish, sense of community, and volunteering (H. L. Smith, Fabricatore, & Peyrot, 1999). Although these instruments are not yet well-established, their existence helps support the argument that important cultural factors affecting both religiosity and, perhaps, health outcomes, may be lost when more global measures are employed.

Health communication scholars examining spirituality in organizations may want to consider denominationally or culture-specific measures such as the ones previously mentioned. For example, in a qualitative study of a Catholic nursing home, Sass (2000) discussed how the concept of organizational spirituality (defined broadly) has not been studied in much depth as of yet. The intersection of spirituality and culture is central to our understanding of the output and impact of religious organizations, especially those providing health services.

Measures of Religious Coping

In contrast to measures of religious belief, many researchers now favor a functionalist approach to the study of RS and health-related variables—relating more than just if an individual engages in religious practices, but how religion helps an individual cope with life stress. Behavioral and communicative responses to health crises may be better predicted by measures of religious coping as opposed to measures of general RS belief (see Sherman & Simonton, 2001). Regarding health outcomes, religious coping has been linked with lowered depression, improved mental and physical health, and reduced mortality (Pargament, Koenig, & Perez, 2000).

Originally, religiosity was included in an instrument measuring 15 possible coping strategies (Carver, Scheier, & Weintraub, 1989). However, researchers now enjoy a much more sophisticated treatment of the specifics of religious coping through the RCOPE (Pargament et al., 2000) and Brief RCOPE (Pargament, Smith, Koenig, & Perez, 1998). The RCOPE is quite comprehensive, including 63 items loading on 17 methods of religious coping. This measure does include both "negative" (attitudes directing an individual away from religiousness) and "positive" coping strategies (attitudes directing an individual toward religiousness as a way to cope). Positive coping strategies include such behaviors as seeking forgiveness of sins, engaging in religious activities to relieve stress, and seeking spiritual support (positive), whereas the negative coping strategies are represented by behaviors such as waiting for God to control the situation, recasting an illness as the work of a demonic force, and viewing illness as punishment from God.

A study of the factor structure of the RCOPE showed that a college student sample provided a reasonable fit for the conceptual factor structure, whereas a sample of elderly medical patients was more strongly supportive (Pargament et al., 1998). Religious coping accounted for unique and significant variance in measures of adjustment when controlling for demographics and measures of global religious belief (Paragment et al., 2000). Specifically, positive coping strategies (e.g., seeking religious support, religious forgiveness and purification) were related to better adjustment, whereas negative coping strategies (e.g., reappraisal of God's powers, spiritual discontentment) were related to poorer adjustment (Pargament et al., 2000).

When the length of the RCOPE makes its administration awkward, the 14-item brief RCOPE may be used (Pargament et al., 1998). This scale includes seven positive religious coping (e.g., "Sought God's love and care") and seven negative religious coping items (e.g., "Wondered what I did for God to punish me"). In tests, the reliability for the brief form ranged from .81 to .91 for positive religious coping, with lower reliabilities (.54 to .70) for negative religious coping. Both RCOPE and Brief RCOPE have been used with diverse samples such as college students, people living with physical and mental illnesses, and people exposed to traumatic events such as the Oklahoma City bombing (Pargament et al., 1998). With words such as *God, church,* and *clergy,* these instruments are best used with Judeo-Christian samples.

These scales of religious coping may be very applicable to health communication studies that focus on communicative processes when dealing with health-related issues, such as message interpretation, the giving and receiving of social support, and coping with illness. In studies where an interaction framework is central, and messages are highlighted, measures of religious coping could provide additional information about how people utilize available resources. For example, entertainment-education, typically grounded in social cognitive theory, can utilize fictional characters to enhance the persuasiveness of health messages (Slater & Rouner, 2002). Just as the similarity of fictional characters to the target audience is important when implementing this type of campaign, RS variables such as how and if the character prays, or otherwise turns to RS to cope with illness, can affect message impact. In addition to this application, coping is already a topic of interest to communication researchers, for example, those who study breast cancer survivors (e.g., Reardon & Buck, 1989; Sullivan, 1997) or bad news delivery (Beach, 2002). Communication research on coping would be remiss if all possible avenues used by individuals were not considered when dealing with health-related events.

Related to religious coping, religious problem-solving scales provide insight into the functional use of religion in overcoming obstacles. The three subscales (*self-directing,* "After I've gone through a rough time, I try to make sense of it without relying on God;" *collaborative,* "When it comes to deciding how to solve a problem, God and I work together as partners"; and *deferring* "Rather than trying to come up with the right solution to a problem myself, I let God decide how to deal with it") represent different ways people take initiative and responsibility versus leaving control to God (Thurston, 1999). The Deferring style is associated with high external rule-based religiosity, whereas the Self-Directing style is more indicative of a quest orientation. The collaborative style is conceptually similar to intrinsic religiosity (Thurston, 1999). The Religious Problem-Solving Scale has shown good internal consistency and test–retest reliability (Pargament et al., 1998) and has been used in diverse samples such as college students, religious groups, recovering alcoholics, and family members in hospital waiting rooms (Pargament et al., 1991; Sherman & Simonton, 2001). Regarding communication research and this instrument, the work of Babrow and colleagues regarding the frameworks of problematic integration and uncertainty management in decision making and health touches these issues as well (e.g., Brashers & Babrow, 1996). How religious problem solving factors into communication and decision making in health contexts could be an exciting new area of study.

Measures of Spiritual Well-Being

Another direction open to researchers is to explore the more existential and universal aspects of RS, such as one's spiritual well-being, defined by Ellison (1983) as "the affirmation of life in a relationship with God, self, community, and environment that nurtures and celebrates wholeness" (p. 330). There are two predominant scales to measure this construct, one that is shorter and has been tested more extensively with medical samples (Paloutzian & Ellison, 1982), and one much longer instrument with 13 related subscales (Moberg, 1984).

The Spiritual Well-Being Scale (SWB) by Paloutzian and Ellison has been called "unquestionably the most widely applied sociopsychometric instrument" (Moberg, 2002, p. 54) on the topic of spirituality. Examples of populations studied include elderly women, people living with cancer or AIDS, religious groups, prison inmates, caregivers for the terminally ill, and medical and psychiatric outpatients (Bufford, Paloutzian, & Ellison, 1991; Ledbetter, Smith, Vosler–Hunter, & Fischer, 1991). The SWB is comprised of 20 items forming two subscales: the Religious Well-Being (RWB) subscale that measures the "vertical" component, or sense of relationship with God, and the Existential Well-Being (EWB) subscale, the "horizontal" component that expresses one's spiritual purpose and satisfaction with life (Ellerhorst–Ryan, 1997). Sample items from the RWB include "My relationship with God helps me not to feel lonely," and "I believe that God loves me and cares about me." Sample items from the EWB include "I feel very fulfilled and satisfied with my life," and "I feel a sense of well-being about the direction my life is headed in." The two subscales have been used together or separately (e.g., Zorn & Johnson, 1997). Particularly popular in nursing research, the instrument has adequate reliability, internal consistency, and construct validity (Boivin, Kirby, Underwood, & Silva, 1999), yet has been questioned regarding its ceiling effects, bias toward Protestant faith over Catholic, and possible three-factor structure instead of the claimed two-factor structure (W. Slater et al., 2001). The scales have been used extensively with clinical samples, including patients coping with anxiety (Kaczorowski, 1989), breast cancer (Mickley, Soeken, & Belcher, 1992), and AIDS (Carson & Green, 1992).

The sheer popularity of the SWB in research related to health outcomes may provide an impetus for health communication scholars to explore this dimension of well-being. Scholars and practitioners are easily convinced that emotional well-being can affect health outcomes, including physical condition. However, the dimension of spirituality has often not been integrated into the biopsychosocial model of health that so many health researchers and clinicians espouse. Mind, body, and spirit are all important components to health, and this measure may be the most reliable and well-tested instrument for assessing RS in health samples in general populations to date.

Other RS Measures of Interest

Some other available scales provide slightly different angles to the empirical study of RS variables: The Systems of Belief Inventory–Revised by Holland et al. (1999) focuses on social factors related to spirituality, a dimension of particular interest to scholars of interpersonal communication and social support. For those looking to include individuals who ascribe to nontheistic religions, the 32-item Mysticism Scale (Hood, 1975) is well-established. This scale focuses on intense singular events that produce feelings of either "oneness" or "nothingness," perhaps apart from religious interpretation (Burris, 1999a; Sherman & Simonton, 2001). On the flip side, an instrument that spotlights ordinary as opposed to extraordinary spiritual experiences, the Daily Spiritual Experience Scale (Underwood & Teresi, 2002), is a newer 16-item instrument testing the experience of awe, joy, and inner peace, and has begun to be used with health-related data in Judeo-Christian samples. Of interest to communication scholars, the Spiritual Assessment Inventory (SAI; Hall & Edwards, 1996) is based on the idea of relationship: that "people relate to God through the same psychological processes and mechanisms with which they relate to other people" (W. Slater et al., 2001, p. 13). The SAI has five dimensions: awareness, instability, defensiveness and disappointment, grandiosity, and realistic acceptance (Hall & Edwards, 1996). Finally, several instruments are available to measure death anxiety, a related construct that has been associated with more physical and psychological problems (see Fortner & Neimeyer, 1999, for a review).

RELIGIOSITY MEASURES IN COMMUNICATION RESEARCH

RS scales are a valuable addition to any study to provide influential demographic information. If researchers believe that information such as a participants' socioeconomic status, race, or gender may contribute to the health behavior or outcome in question, then surely RS beliefs and practices should be assessed as well. This final section is designed to provide health communication researchers with some ideas for how RS variables can be incorporated into a few of the most popular lines of research. Although our intention here is just to provide a few ideas for future studies, clearly, there is a host of other ways in which RS variables could be integrated into our research programs.

One fundamental way in which RS affects individuals is through identity and sense of self. Blaine, Trivedi, and Eshleman (1998) argued that "religion should be recognized as a prominent and potentially robust sociocultural influence on the self-concept that shapes the way people think about and describe themselves" (p. 1041). Due to its centrality in the provider–patient relationship and the effectiveness of medical interviewing, how people describe themselves (e.g., self-disclosure) is a topic of interest for health communication researchers (e.g., Duggan & Parrott, 2001; Robinson, 1998). Self-disclosure is also an important topic for researchers interested in communication about sexual interactions (e.g., Brown & Basil, 1995; Lucchetti, 1999). There is much to be learned about how communication within a religious group affects one's self-concept regarding health and how RS variables might affect willingness to disclose health-related information to a health care provider or to a romantic partner.

Related to the idea of self-concept is another popular construct for health communication campaign designers: self-efficacy. Witte's (1992, 1994) work with fear appeals has shown how self-efficacy, or the feeling that one is capable of performing a desired response, is instrumental to the effectiveness of health messages containing risk components. As self-efficacy is key to successful health campaign message construction (Witte, Meyer, & Martell, 2001), health campaign designers should not only consider how self-efficacy affects message acceptance, but how messages can be designed to promote self-efficacy (Egbert & Parrott, 2001). RS instruments such as religious coping, decision making, and spiritual well-being may become helpful tools when investigating these topics.

Hamilton and Rubin (1992) found that religiosity affected television viewing in that more religious people were less interested in viewing programs with sexual content and watched television less. In health communication, the concept of "sensation seeking," or the proclivity for intense, graphic, and arousing messages, is linked to drug use; teens and young adults who are high sensation seekers are more likely to attend to antidrug messages with high sensation value (Palmgreen, Donohew, & Harrington, 2001). Based on these two conclusions, it would be beneficial to learn about the characteristics of religious populations with regard to sensation seeking: Do health messages with low sensation value appeal more to religious or spiritual teens and young adults, or is there little difference with regard to RS variables?

There are countless outlets for scholars of social support to use one or more of the RS instruments reviewed here. Researchers who employ network analyses should take careful note of the differences between intrinsic and extrinsic religiosity to learn more about how RS variables affect social support through either membership in a social network or through the spiritual relationship itself. Actual interactions could be highlighted to learn more about the content of social support with regard to health topics: How do religious groups use communication to maintain social norms with regard to health issues? Is there evidence of negative support that affects individuals' coping during and after health crises?

Ethical Issues and Warnings

Although research using RS variables might be considered ethereal, and therefore above more practical considerations, it is still subject to the same ethical principles of conduct as with any other empirical line of study. Some question has arisen concerning the appropriateness of employing RS variables if the participant is under stress and is therefore considered vulnerable. However, numerous studies have been conducted with participants in vulnerable situations and have provided valuable information while still protecting participant rights. Foremost among these protection mechanisms is review by an institutional review board or formal research review committee. A good example of managing ethical considerations in research on hospice patients, long considered a vulnerable population, has been provided by Casarett et al. (2001), who recommended that researchers pay more attention to the "structural sources" of ethical challenges (things such as assessing the risks and benefits of the research, providing basic education in research ethics to the staff, addressing short length of stay, and assessing demands of research projects on participants' resources and personnel needs). Researchers who include RS variables should exercise caution to help ensure that their research will not trigger undue concern or uncertainty, especially when also asking questions regarding participants' health status.

Another concern that arises with RS variables is how to explain outlying scores. A conservative approach should be used in interpreting scores for those who do not fit in with majority opinion or belief. Moberg (2002) warned of prejudice and discrimination that can result from classifying scores from devout minority religious groups with deviants or outliers. Whether these individuals are classified as cultists (outside a mainstream religious denomination) or simply devout believers depends on the researcher's discretion and careful framing of the situation under consideration. This concern again points to the importance of using multidimensional measures to capture the complex nature of religious belief and behavior, as study results may be open to discriminatory interpretation.

Regarding the interplay of culture and RS variables, Guttman (1997) reminded us to respect participants' values, even if they differ from the values the campaign is advocating. She instructed educators that what might be a health problem from their perspective might be a desired state from the perspective of the participant, and warns educators against using dependent variables, such as RS values, in a manipulative manner to change participants in ways desired by the educator, but not necessarily by the participants themselves. As authors, we too encourage the readers of this article to use the RS norms and worldviews discussed earlier in a way that shows respect for the learner or research participant rather than to advance their own agendas.

Finally, we would like to leave the reader with a few warnings related to the use of RS scales in health communication research. As with any tool, these measures carry inherent strengths and weaknesses. Used appropriately and heeding the following suggestions, we believe that careful consideration of RS variables in empirical research may add a great deal to health communication studies:

1. Carefully investigate how RS scales may overlap with various demographic variables such as gender and education.

2. Consider the psychometrics of any instrument, including sensitivity, reliability, and validity. Multi-item measures are preferable (Koenig et al., 2001).
3. Have a clear conceptualization of the construct and its related measurement. Each scale has a slightly different angle for assessing RS (Hill et al., 1998).
4. Watch logistics of scales; measures vary in readability, length, and so forth (Hill & Hood, 1999).
5. Decide whether specific or global measures are needed (Moberg, 2002).
6. Beware of definitional issues regarding religiosity, spirituality, and God (Koenig et al, 2001).
7. Consider alternatives to cross-sectional studies and self-report health indicators (the overuse of these is a common criticism of RS research).

CONCLUSIONS

Levin (1994) summed up the charge for health communication scholars: "Finally, little attention has been given to delineating the clinical and public health applications of these findings" (p. 1481). Much attention has been paid to the psychological relations between various RS and other psychological constructs, but few studies investigate how RS functions to alleviate health problems. Health communication scholars are in a unique position to lend their expertise to questions such as how religious commitment can be used in constructing persuasive health messages, and how a relationship with God can affect the strength and quality of social support networks during times of stress or illness. There are already over 100 RS scales in existence (Hill & Hood, 1999). Health communication researchers can use the existing psychometric literature available about many of these scales to immediately begin including these important constructs in our research. In addition to these quantitative tools, qualitative scholars can expand on the RS linkages to health outcomes through methodologies such as interviews, focus groups, and ethnographies. There are numerous possible sources of funding for new research projects linking health with RS variables.[1] In addition, interested readers are referred to the commis-

---

[1]Agencies that have funded projects investigating religiosity and spirituality variables and health include the National Institutes of Health (www.nih.gov), specifically the National Cancer Institute, the National Center for Complementary and Alternative Medicine, the National Heart, Lung, and Blood Institute, the National Human Genome Research Institute, the National Institute of Mental Health, the National Institute of Nursing Research, the National Institute on Aging, the National Institute on Alcohol Abuse and Alcoholism, and the National Institute on Drug Abuse. Other funding agencies include Pew Charitable Trusts (http://www.pewtrusts.com/grants/), the John S. and James L Knight Foundation (http://www.dsacommunityfoundation.com/grant-making/), and the Lilly Endowment (http://www.lilly.com/about/community/foundation/endowment.html).

sioned National Institute for Healthcare Research report (Larson et al., 1998), which contains many suggestions and resources for research in this area. As religion and spirituality continue to be central to at least half of the population of North America, social scientists and communication scholars cannot afford to continue our dormant state with regard to its influence on health communication and health outcomes.

ACKNOWLEDGMENT

This article was previously presented as a paper to the Health Communication Division of the National Communication Association, November 24, 2002.

REFERENCES

Adamson, G., Shevlin, M., Lloyd, N. S. V., & Lewis, C. A. (2000). An integrated approach for assessing reliability and validity: An application of structural equation modeling to the measurement of religiosity. *Personality and Individual Differences, 29,* 971–979.

Allport, G. W., & Ross, J. M. (1967). Personal religious orientation and prejudice. *Journal of Personality and Social Psychology, 5,* 432–443.

Babrow, A. S. (1992). Communication and problematic integration: Understanding diverging probability and value, ambiguity, ambivalence, and impossibility. *Communication Theory, 2,* 95–130.

Babrow, A. S., Hines, S. C., & Kasch, C. R. (2000). Managing uncertainty in illness explanation: An application of problematic integration theory. In B. B. Whaley (Ed.), *Explaining illness: Messages, strategies, and contexts* (pp. 41–67). Mahwah, NJ: Lawrence Erlbaum Associates, Inc.

Bassett, R. L. (1999). Intrinsic religious motivation scale. In P. C. Hill & R. W. Hood (Eds.), *Measures of religiosity* (pp. 135–137). Birmingham, AL: Religious Education Press.

Batson, C. D., & Schoenrade, P. (1991a). Measuring religion as quest I. Validity concerns. *Journal for the Scientific Study of Religion, 30,* 416–429.

Batson, C. D., & Schoenrade, P. (1991b). Measuring religion as quest: II. Reliability concerns. *Journal for the Scientific Study of Religion, 30,* 430–447.

Beach, W. A. (2002). Between dad and son: Initiating, delivering, and assimilating bad cancer news. *Health Communication, 14,* 271–298.

Benson, P. L., Dehority, J., Garman, L., Hanson, E., Hochschwender, M., Lebold, C., et al. (1980). Interpersonal correlates of non-spontaneous helping behavior. *Journal of Social Psychology, 110,* 87–95.

Blaine, B. E., Trivedi, P., & Eshleman, A. (1998). Religious belief and the self–concept: Evaluating the implications for psychological adjustment. *Personality and Social Psychology Bulletin, 24,* 1040–1052.

Boivin, M. J., Kirby, A. L., Underwood, L. K., & Silva, H. (1999). Spiritual well-being scale. In P. C. Hill & R. W. Hood (Eds.), *Measures of religiosity* (pp. 382–385). Birmingham, AL: Religious Education Press.

Brashers, D. E., & Babrow, A. S. (1996). Theorizing communication and health. *Communication Studies, 47,* 243–252.

Brashers, D. E., Neidig, J. L., Haas, S. M., Dobbs, L. K., Cardillo, L. W., & Russell, J. A. (2000). Communication in the management of uncertainty: The case of persons living with HIV or AIDS. *Communication Monographs, 67,* 63–84.

Brown, W. J., & Basil, M. D. (1995). Media celebrities and public health: Responses to "Magic" Johnson's HIV disclosure and its impact on AIDS risk and high-risk behaviors. *Health Communication, 7,* 345–370.

Bufford, R. K., Paloutzian, R. F., & Ellison, C. W. (1991). Norms for the spiritual well-being scale. *Journal of Psychology and Theology, 19,* 56–70.

Burleson, B. R. (1983). Social cognition, empathic motivation, and adults' comforting strategies. *Human Communication Research, 10,* 295–304.

Burris, C. T. (1999a). The mysticism scale: Research form D (M scale). In P. C. Hill & R. W. Hood (Eds.), *Measures of religiosity* (pp. 363–367). Birmingham, AL: Religious Education Press.

Burris, C. T. (1999b). Religious orientation scale. In P. C. Hill & R. W. Hood (Eds.), *Measures of religiosity* (pp. 144–154). Birmingham, AL: Religious Education Press.

Carballo, M. (n.d.). *Religion in the world at the end of the millennium.* Retrieved July 26, 2002, from http://www.gallup–international.com

Carson, V. B., & Green, H. (1992). Spiritual well-being: A predictor of hardiness in patients with acquired immunodeficiency syndrome. *Journal of Professional Nursing, 8,* 209–220.

Carver, C. S., Scheier, M. E., & Weintraub, J. K. (1989). Assessing coping strategies: A theoretically based approach. *Journal of Personality and Social Psychology, 56,* 267–283.

Casarett, D., Ferrell, B., Kirschling, J., Levetown, M., Merriman, M. P., Ramey, M., et al. (2001). NHPCO Task Force statement on the ethics of hospice participation in research. *Journal of Palliative Medicine, 4,* 441–449.

Conn, M. K., & Peterson, C. (1989). Social support: Seek and ye shall find. *Journal of Social and Personal Relationships, 6,* 345–358.

Donahue, M. J. (1985). Intrinsic and extrinsic religiousness: Review and meta-analysis. *Journal of Personality and Social Psychology, 48,* 400–419.

Duggan, A. P., & Parrott, R. L. (2001). Physicians' nonverbal rapport building and patients' talk about the subjective component of illness. *Human Communication Research, 27,* 299–311.

Egbert, N., & Parrott, R. (2001). Self-efficacy and rural women's performance of breast and cervical cancer detection practices. *Journal of Health Communication, 6,* 219–233.

Ellerhorst–Ryan, J. M. (1997). Instruments to measure aspects of spirituality. In M. Frank–Stromborg & S. J. Olsen (Eds.), *Instruments for clinical health-care research* (2nd ed., pp. 202–212). Boston: Jones and Bartlett Publishers.

Ellison, C. W. (1983). Spiritual well-being: Conceptualization and measurement. *Journal of Psychology & Theology, 11,* 330–340.

Fortner, B. V., & Neimeyer, R. A. (1999). Death anxiety in older adults: A quantitative review. *Death Studies, 23,* 387–411.

Francis, L. J., & Stubbs, M. T. (1987). Measuring attitudes toward Christianity: From childhood to adulthood. *Personality and Individual Differences, 8,* 741–743.

Gorsuch, R. L., & Venable, G. D. (1983). Development of an "age universal" I–E scale. *Journal for the Scientific Study of Religion, 22,* 181–187.

Guttman, N. (1997). Beyond strategic research: A value-centered approach to health communication interventions. *Communication Theory, 7,* 95–124.

Hall, T. W., & Edwards, K. J. (1996). The initial development and factor analysis of the spiritual assessment inventory. *Journal of Psychology and Theology, 24,* 233–246.

Hamilton, N. F., & Rubin, A. M. (1992). The influence of religiosity on television viewing. *Journalism Quarterly, 6,* 667–678.

Hill, P. C. (1999). Age universal religious orientation scale. In P. C. Hill & R. W. Hood (Eds.), *Measures of religiosity* (pp. 121–123). Birmingham, AL: Religious Education Press.

Hill, P. C., & Hood, R. W. (Eds.). (1999). *Measures of religiosity.* Birmingham, AL: Religious Education Press.

Hill, P. C., Pargament, K. I., Swyers, J. P., Gorsuch, R. L., McCullough, M. E., Hood, R. W., et al. (1998). Definitions of religion and spirituality. In D. B. Larson, J. P. Swyers, & M. E. McCullough (Eds.), *Scientific research on spirituality and health: A consensus report* (pp. 14–31). Rockville, MD: National Institute for Healthcare Research.

Hinebaugh-Igoe, L. (1999). Index of core spiritual experiences. In P. C. Hill & R. W. Hood (Eds.), *Measures of religiosity* (pp. 360–363). Birmingham, AL: Religious Education Press.

Hoge, D. R. (1972). A validated intrinsic religious motivation scale. *Journal for the Scientific Study of Religion, 11,* 369–376.

Holland, J. C., Passik, S., Kash, K. M., Russak, S. M., Gronert, M. K., Sison, A., et al. (1999). The role of religious and spiritual beliefs in coping with malignant melanoma. *Psycho-Oncology, 8,* 14–26.

Hood, R. W. (1975). The construction and preliminary validation of a measure of reported mystical experience. *Journal for the Scientific Study of Religion, 14,* 29–41.

Hunsberger, B. (1996). Religious fundamentalism, right-wing authoritarianism, and hostility toward homosexuals in non-Christian religious groups. *International Journal for the Psychology of Religion, 6,* 39–49.

Jagers, R. J., & Smith, P. (1996). Further examination of the spirituality scale. *Journal of Black Psychology, 22,* 429–442.

Kaczorowski, J. M. (1989). Spiritual well-being and anxiety in adults diagnosed with cancer. *The Hospice Journal, 5,* 105–115.

Kass, J. D., Friedman, R., Lesserman, J., Zuttermeister, P., & Benson, H. (1991). Health outcomes and a new index of spiritual experience. *Journal for the Scientific Study of Religion, 30,* 203–211.

Kirkpatrick, L. A., & Hood, R. W., Jr. (1990). Intrinsic–extrinsic religious orientation: The boon or bane of contemporary psychology of religion? *Journal for the Scientific Study of Religion, 29,* 442–462.

Kirkwood, W. G. (1994). Studying communication about spirituality and the spiritual consequences of communication. *The Journal of Communication and Religion, 17,* 13–26.

Koenig, H. G., George, L. K., Cohen, H. J., Hays, J. C., Blazer, D. G., & Larson, D. B. (1998). The relationship between religious activities and blood pressure in older adults. *International Journal of Psychiatry in Medicine, 28,* 189–213.

Koenig, H. G., McCullough, M. E., & Larson, D. B. (2001). *Handbook of religion and health.* New York: Oxford University Press.

Koenig, H. G., Meador, K., & Parkerson, G. (1997). Religion index for psychiatric research: A 5-item measure for use in health outcomes studies [Letter to the Editor]. *American Journal of Psychiatry, 154,* 885–886.

Larimore, W. L., Parker, M., & Crowther, M. (2002). Should clinicians incorporate positive spirituality into their practices? What does the evidence say? *Annals of Behavioral Medicine, 24,* 69–73.

Larson, D. B., Swyers, J. P., & McCullough, M. E. (Eds.). (1998). *Scientific research on spirituality and health: A consensus report.* Rockville, MD: National Institute for Healthcare Research.

Ledbetter, M. F., Smith, L. A., Vosler–Hunter, W. L., & Fischer, J. D. (1991). An evaluation of the research and clinical usefulness of the Spiritual Well-Being Scale. *Journal of Psychology and Theology, 19,* 49–55.

Levin, J. S. (1994). Religion and health: Is there an association, is it valid, and is it causal? *Social Science and Medicine, 38,* 1475–1482.

Lewis, C. A., Shevlin, M., McGuckin, C., & Navratil, M. (2001). The Santa Clara strength of religious faith questionnaire: Confirmatory factor analysis. *Pastoral Psychology, 49,* 379–384.

Lipkus, I. M. (2001). Informing women about their breast cancer risks: Truth and consequences. *Health Communication, 12,* 205–227.

Lucchetti, A. E. (1999). Deception in disclosing one's sexual history: Safe-sex avoidance or ignorance? *Communication Quarterly, 47,* 300–314.

Lukwago, S. N., Bucholtz, D. C., Kreuter, M. W., Holt, C. L., & Clark, E. M. (2001). Development and validation of brief scales to measure collectivism, religiosity, racial pride, and time orientation in urban African American women. *Family and Community Health, 24,* 63–71.

Maltby, J. (1999). Religious orientation and Eysenck's personality dimensions: The use of the amended religious orientation scale to examine the relationship between religiosity, psychoticism, neuroticism, and extraversion. *Personality and Individual Differences, 26,* 79–84.

Maltby, J., & Day, L. (1998). Amending a measure of the Quest Religious Orientation: Applicability of the scale's use among religious and non-religious persons. *Personality and Individual Differences, 25,* 517–522.

Maltby, J., & Lewis, C. A. (1996). Measuring intrinsic and extrinsic orientation toward religion: Amendments for its use among religious and non-religious samples. *Personality and Individual Differences, 21,* 937–946.

Maltby, J., & Lewis, C. A. (1997). The reliability and validity of a short scale of attitude towards Christianity among U.S.A., English, Republic of Ireland, and Northern Ireland adults. *Personality and Individual Differences, 22,* 649–654.

Mickley, J. R., Soeken, K., & Belcher, A. (1992). Spiritual well-being, religiousness and hope among women with breast cancer. *IMAGE: Journal of Nursing Scholarship, 24,* 267–272.

Miller, J. K. (2002). Beyond the organ donor card: The effect of knowledge, attitudes, and values on willingness to communicate about organ donation to family members. *Health Communication, 14,* 121–135.

Moberg, D. O. (1984). Subjective measures of spiritual well-being. *Review of Religious Research, 25,* 351–359.

Moberg, D. O. (2002). Assessing and measuring spirituality: Confronting dilemmas of universal and particular evaluative criteria. *Journal of Adult Development, 9,* 47–60.

Morgan. S. E., & Miller, J. K. (2002). Communicating about gifts of life: The effect of knowledge, attitudes, and altruism on behavior and behavioral intentions regarding organ donation. *Journal of Applied Communication Research, 30*(2), 163–179.

Nelson, P. B. (1989). Ethnic differences in intrinsic/extrinsic religious orientation and depression in the elderly. *Archives of Psychiatric Nursing, 3,* 199–204.

Palmgreen, P., Donohew, L., & Harrington, N. G. (2001). Sensation seeking in antidrug campaign and message design. In R. E. Rice & C. K. Atkin (Eds.), *Public communication campaigns* (3rd ed., pp. 300–304). Thousand Oaks, CA: Sage.

Paloutzian, R. F., & Ellison, C. W. (1982). Loneliness, spiritual well-being and quality of life. In L. A. Peplau & D. Perlman (Eds.), *Loneliness: A sourcebook of current theory, research and therapy* (pp. 224–237). New York: Wiley-Interscience.

Paloutzian, R. F., & Kirkpatrick, L. A. (1995). Introduction: The scope of religious influences on personal and societal well-being. *Journal of Social Issues, 51*(2), 1–11.

Pargament, K. I., Falgout, K., Ensing, D. S., Reilly, B., Silverman, M., Van Haitsma, K., et al. (1991). The congregational development program: Data-based consultation with churches and synagogues. *Professional Psychology: Research and Practice, 22,* 393–404.

Pargament, K. I., Koenig, H. G., & Perez, L. M. (2000). The many methods of religious coping: Development and initial validation of the RCOPE. *Journal of Clinical Psychology, 56,* 519–543.

Pargament, K. I., Olson, H., Reilly, B., Falgout, K., Ensing, D. S., & Van Haitsma, K. (1992). God help me (II): The relationship of religious orientations to religious coping with negative life events. *Journal for the Scientific Study of Religion, 31,* 504–513.

Pargament, K. I., & Park, C. L. (1995). Merely a defense? The variety of religious means and ends. *Journal of Social Issues, 51*(2), 15–32.

Pargament, K. I., Smith, B. W., Koenig, H. G., & Perez, L. (1998). Patterns of positive and negative religious coping with negative life stressors. *Journal for the Scientific Study of Religion, 37,* 710–724.

Plante, T. G., & Sherman, A. C. (Eds.). (2001). *Faith and health: Psychological perspectives.* New York: Guilford.

Query, J. L., & Kreps, G. L. (1996). Testing a relational model for health communication competence among caregivers for individuals with Alzheimer's disease. *Journal of Health Psychology, 1,* 335–351.

Reardon, K. K., & Buck, R. (1989). Emotion, reason, and communication in coping with cancer. *Health Communication, 1,* 41–55.

Robinson, J. D. (1998). Getting down to business: Talk, gaze, and body orientation during openings of doctor–patient consultations. *Human Communication Research, 25,* 97–123.

Sass, J. S. (2000). Characterizing organizational spirituality: A communication culture approach. *Communication Studies, 51,* 40–51.

Sherman, A. C., Plante, T. G., Simonton, S., Adams, D. C., Harbison, C., & Burris, S. K. (2000). A multidimensional measure of religious involvement for cancer patients: The Duke Religious Index. *Journal of Supportive Care in Cancer, 8,* 102–109.

Sherman, A. C., & Simonton, S. (2001). Assessment of religiousness and spirituality in health research. In T. G. Plante & A. C. Sherman (Eds.), *Faith and health: Psychological perspectives* (pp. 139–163). New York: Guilford.

Slater, M., & Rouner, D. (2002). Entertainment-education and elaboration likelihood: Understanding the processing of narrative persuasion. *Communication Theory, 12,* 173–191.

Slater, W., Hall, T. W., & Edwards, K. J. (2001). Measuring religion and spirituality: Where are we and where are we going? *Journal of Psychology and Theology, 29,* 4–21.

Sloan, R. P., & Bagiella, E. (2002). Claims about religious involvement and health outcomes. *Annals of Behavioral Medicine, 24,* 14–21.

Smith, H. L., Fabricatore, A., & Peyrot, M. (1999). Religiosity and altruism among African American males: The Catholic experience. *Journal of Black Studies, 29,* 579–597.

Smith, T. W. (2001). Religion and spirituality in the science and practice of health psychology. In T. G. Plante & A. C. Sherman (Eds.), *Faith and health: Psychological perspectives* (pp. 355–380). New York: Guilford.

Sullivan, C. F. (1997). Women's ways of coping with breast cancer. *Women's Studies in Communication, 20,* 59–82.

Thoresen, C. E., & Harris, A. H. (2002). Spirituality and health: What's the evidence and what's needed? *Annals of Behavioral Medicine, 24,* 3–13.

Thoresen, C. E., Harris, A. H., & Oman, D. (2001). Spirituality, religion, and health: Evidence, issues, and concerns. In T. G. Plante & A. C. Sherman (Eds.), *Faith and health: Psychological perspectives* (pp. 15–52). New York: Guilford.

Thurston, N. S. (1999). Religious problem-solving scale. In P. C. Hill & R. W. Hood (Eds.), *Measures of religiosity* (pp. 337–350). Birmingham, AL: Religious Education Press.

Underwood, L. G., & Teresi, J. A. (2002). The daily spiritual experience scale: Development, theoretical description, reliability, exploratory factor analysis, and preliminary construct validity using health-related data. *Annals of Behavioral Medicine, 24,* 22–33.

VandeCreek, L., Ayres, S., & Bassham, M. (1995). Using INSPIRIT to conduct spiritual assessments. *Journal of Pastoral Care, 49,* 83–89.

Vishwanath, K., Kahn, E., Finnegan, J. R., Hertog, J., & Potter, J. D. (1993). Motivation and the knowledge gap. *Communication Research, 20,* 546–563.

Witte, K. (1992). Putting the fear back into fear appeals: The extended parallel process model. *Communication Monographs, 59,* 329–349.

Witte, K. (1994). Fear control and danger control: A test of the extended parallel process model (EPPM). *Communication Monographs, 61,* 113–133.

Witte, K., Meyer, G., & Martell, D. (2001). *Effective health risk messages: A step-by-step guide.* Thousand Oaks, CA: Sage.

Zinnbauer, B. J, Pargament, K. I., & Scott, A. B. (1999). The emerging meanings of religiousness and spirituality: Problems and prospects. *Journal of Personality, 67,* 889–919.

Zorn, C. R., & Johnson, M. T. (1997). Religious well-being in noninstitutionalized elderly women. *Health Care for Women International, 18,* 209–219.

HEALTH COMMUNICATION, *16*(1), 29–45

Behavioral Health Outcomes Associated With Religious Faith and Media Exposure About Human Genetics

Roxanne Parrott
Department of Communication Arts & Sciences
The Pennsylvania State University

Kami Silk
Department of Communication
Michigan State University

Janice Raup Krieger
Department of Communication Arts & Sciences
The Pennsylvania State University

Tina Harris and Celeste Condit
Department of Speech Communication
University of Georgia

A number of scholars have speculated that religious people will be less likely than others to ascribe either fatalistic or deterministic powers to genes, opting instead to leave freedom as a choice for both God and humans. This research investigates the role of religious faith (RF) on behavioral health outcomes associated with information about genes and health, as well as its role as a gatekeeper to media information about genes and health. This research is based on the results of a survey of 858 members of the lay public, including northeastern and southeastern rural and urban participants. Findings are considered within frameworks of audience segmentation principles associated with RF.

Requests for reprints should be sent to Roxanne Parrott, The Pennsylvania State University, Department of Communication Arts & Sciences, University Park, PA 16802. E-mail: rlp18@psu.edu

With the mapping of the human genome marking a great scientific achievement, the role of genes in health has assumed prominence in discourse about health promotion and disease prevention (Collins & McKusick, 2001). Genes constitute an invisible contributor (Kundrat & Nussbaum, 2003) to the health equation, introducing unique societal and personal dimensions to debates about how, when, and why health afflictions occur. In the face of the seemingly inexplicable, such as the role of genes in health, some people rely on religious faith (RF) to guide their knowledge and outcome expectancies. RF refers to the predisposition to think, feel, or act based on his or her belief in a spiritual power greater than humans to affect the course of nature and the role of humans within that realm. Extrinsic religiosity, the outward and visible signs and practices associated with RF that include prayer and worship, provides solace, distraction, sociability, and even self-justification (Genia, 1993). Intrinsic religiosity, the internalized expressions and integrated experiences of RF sometimes referred to as spirituality, has been found to be used by the sick and disabled for coping (Genia, 1993). This research investigates the role of RF on behavioral health outcomes associated with information about genes and health, and its role as gatekeeper to media information about genes and health.

RELIGIOUS FAITH AND BEHAVIORAL OUTCOMES

A substantial body of evidence includes references to the role of RF as a social and personal resource for health (e.g., Koenig & Larson, 1998). Extrinsic religiosity functions as a social resource that provides information or assistance through direct communication or vicarious observation (Genia, 1993). Thus, extrinsic religiosity may impact individual beliefs about the role of genes in health based on exposure to the opinions and experiences of faith-based leaders and community members. Intrinsic religiosity functions as a personal resource associated with cognitive and emotional functioning (Dossey, 1993) and may thus provide a coping mechanism in association with information about genes and health. RF is absent in behavioral-health models, however, a conclusion highlighted in previous research (Ashing-Giwa, 1999). This research advances an exploratory model associated with RF and a number of outcomes associated with health communication about genes and health.

Knowledge

Knowledge about genes and health has increased at a rapid pace over the past decade, challenging clinicians to keep pace (Collins & McKusick, 2001), let alone the lay public (Ogamdi, 1994). Important components of such knowledge relate to the mutability of genes associated with the role of environments and personal behavior on genetic expression and health outcomes. For example, any amount of alcohol consumption may impact genetic expression (Bachtell, Wang, Freeman, & Risinger, 1999). Evidence also associates RF with lower incidence of excessive alcohol use, smoking, and sexual experimentation (Levin & Schiller, 1987). The relation between RF and knowledge about how these behaviors relate to genetic expression, however, has not been considered. Knowledge about genetics is related to science literacy, one component of health literacy, defined as the motivation and skills to access and use health information and resources to promote one's health (Christensen & Griffiths, 2000). High levels of RF have been found to be related to low levels of science literacy (Miller, 1983). Knowledge about human genetics relates not only to one's science literacy but also to family history and personal experiences. This suggests that RF may not be related directly to knowledge about genes and health, as illustrated in Figure 1, although knowledge likely impacts directly two other behavioral health outcomes associated with human genetics: self-efficacy and response efficacy.

Self-Efficacy

One of the most significant outcomes of individual knowledge is one's confidence in the ability to gain and maintain control over inputs to a particular behavior, referred to as self-efficacy (Bandura, 1997). Health communicators have ample theory and research implicating the significance of self-efficacy for health beliefs and behaviors (e.g., Egbert & Parrott, 2001). In summarizing predictors of self-efficacy, Bandura included verbal persuasion, vicarious experience, actual experience, physiological and affective states, and the integration of these sources of efficacy information, which often conflict (Bandura, 1997). The role of RF for self-efficacy has not been systematically examined, with the terms *religion, faith,* and *spirituality* absent from the index and discussion in Bandura's volume that summarizes the status of knowledge about self-efficacy. Church attendance, or extrinsic religiosity, has been found to impact perceptions of mastery (Krause & Tran, 1989), perhaps a result of utilizing the faith community as a source of social support (Pargament, 1998), including testimonials, prayer requests, and anointing as health resources (Simpson & King, 1999). RF comprises a source of verbal persuasion, contributing to the availability and accessibility of vicarious and actual experiences as well as physiological and affective states. This suggests that RF may directly impact perceptions of self-efficacy, as illustrated in Figure 1.

Response Efficacy

The mapping of the human genome presents numerous opportunities for science to suggest new avenues for genetic engineering, technologies, and treatments (Khoury, 1996). As a result of information about human genetic research (HGR) being disseminated to the public, expectations relating to the availability and ef-

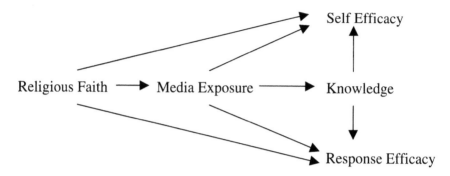

FIGURE 1   The theoretical relation among religion, media, and behavioral health outcomes.

fectiveness of genetic engineering and treatments, or response efficacy, may outdistance the availability of these technologies and therapies. Scholars have speculated that religious people will be less likely than others to ascribe either fatalistic or deterministic powers to genes, opting instead to leave freedom as a choice for both God and humans (Kerr, Cunningham-Burley, & Amos, 1998). However, intrinsic religiosity provides a guide for moral judgments, suggesting what is good and bad behavior (Clark & Dawson, 1996). Many organized religions have taken formal positions against human cloning, for example, which may impact individual attitudes regarding HGR. As with self-efficacy, RF appears likely to impact directly the formation of perceptions associated with response efficacy and human genetics, as illustrated in Figure 1. An examination of the role of religiosity on the lay public's outcome expectancies may guide the planning of health communication associated with this topic, as well as the evolution of behavioral health models:

RQ1:   Does (1) intrinsic or (2) extrinsic religiosity relate to (a) knowledge, (b) self-efficacy, or (c) response efficacy associated with human genetics and health?

RELIGIOUS FAITH AND MEDIA USE

Media comprises an important means of disseminating health information through strategic health promotion (Salmon & Atkin, 2003), popular entertainment, and a hybrid of the two in the form of entertainment-education (Kline, 2003). Consideration of when media content is used comprises one domain of media effects theory and research. Of necessity, understanding why some media appear to have greater or lesser effects requires consideration of exposure to media. Oliver (2002) advanced two overarching explanations for media effects: (a) enjoyment and emotional response and (b) selective exposure, interpretation, and memory. Each explanation affords a framework for understanding how RF may impact individual media use. As the genre of religious programming on television gained prominence in the 1980s, research affirmed that individuals watched because they regarded content on nonreligious television to be morally offensive, a reactionary viewing pattern (Abelman, 1987; Abelman & Hoover, 1990; Gerbner, Gross, Hoover, Morgan, & Signorielli, 1984). Research suggests that little has changed regarding content, as viewers encounter violence in two out of three programs viewed on TV (Smith, Nathanson, & Wilson, 2002). The potential of RF to impact use of multiple media modalities with relations to genetics and health has both theoretic and pragmatic importance.

Movies

Films have long portrayed the role of genes on human beings but with varied plot lines. Portrayal associated with evil children, illustrated by such movies as *The Bad Seed,* locates evil in the child as an inherited condition rather than a response to parenting or society. This mid-20th century novel turned film portrayed violence as a characteristic that runs in the main character's blood, so it cannot be exorcised, a eugenic theory of pollution (Jackson, 2000). At the end of the 20th century, however, movies blurred the lines between actual and potential achievements in story lines such as Columbia Pictures science fiction story, *Gattaca* (1997), in which the potential for genetic engineering to determine individual futures is contested. Whether RF impacts individual exposure patterns associated with such films, an extension of the reactionary viewing pattern associated with avoidance of secular TV, has seldom been considered. Moreover, despite the decades of movie entertainment containing such messages, their impact on behavioral health outcomes has been neglected. The findings observed with regard to entertainment TV and health more broadly, especially for younger audiences where involvement and interest in health information is less (O'Keefe, Boyd, & Brown, 1998), suggest that movies may be influential in such domains.

Daytime Televised Talk Shows

Little attention has been paid to talk shows as a focus of research associated with exposure to health information despite the fact that drug abuse and teen pregnancy, for example, are topics often discussed on talk shows (Davis & Mares, 2002). Talk show hosts range from Oprah Winfrey to Jerry Springer, reflecting a broad range in topics and guests (Bernstein, 1994; Priest, 1995). It has been observed that "political officials enlist talk-show hosts of similar ideological persuasion to mobilize public support for their legislative initiatives and opposition to those they dislike" (Bandura, 1997, p. 492). Among these initiatives may be references to stem cell research and other human genetics scientific endeavors. The lay public may gain some knowledge about human genetics research as a result of exposure to talk shows that address these issues.

Whether RF impacts the likelihood of exposure to talk shows is not known, but the press has characterized talk show guests and viewing audiences as immoral (Birmingham, 2000). Although some talk shows may be considered to consist of extreme examples of immoral behavior and judgments, others may showcase humanity at its best. One study of the prime time show, *Married with Children,* for example, found that one of the main female characters, Peggy Bundy, watched talk shows as a strategy of empowerment, a means to gain access to a world beyond her experience, with particular identification with Oprah Winfrey (Lusanne, 1999). Talk show content is often characterized by narrow, conservative, mainstream values associated with a White, middle class, male dominant culture, in which women have a specific traditional place and role (Birmingham, 2000). Such content, as exemplified by the *Jerry Springer Show,* functions as moralizing rituals (Grabe, 2002). Whether this relates to knowledge and efficacy perceptions about HGR, as compared to specific issues such as cloning, is debatable.

Prime Time Medical and Crime Shows

Termed "the dominant form of mass media" (Vanderford, 1999, p. 33), television provides a ubiquitous medium through which lessons about life, including health and the relation of genes to human traits including health, may be learned. Medical dramas, including *Marcus Welby, M.D., Trapper John, St. Elsewhere, Chicago Hope, ER,* and *LA Doctors,* have been a mainstay of prime time TV. A content analysis of two seasons of *ER* and *Chicago Hope* revealed an emphasis on the use of technology in healing (Harter & Japp, 2001), suggesting that exposure to these shows may increase perceptions of and expectations for genetic enhancements and technologies associated with perceptions of response efficacy. The impact of RF on exposure to prime time TV that includes information about human genetics may be negative, as some RF organizations explicitly review content and make recommendations associated with media exposure. "Focus on the Family," a nonprofit, Christian-centered organization started in 1977 as a response to Dr. James Dobson's increasing concern for the American family, for example, posts reviews of TV, movies, and music on its Web site. These include *CSI: Crime Scene Investigation* (Isaac, 2001), with the review asking, "Should families entertain themselves by ingesting graphic images of medical autopsies, brutalized bodies, blood-spattered sets and decomposing corpses?" and asserting that, "CSI is ugly, exploitative, gross, disrespectful of the dead and, unfortunately, enormously popular among the living" (Isaac,

2001). RF may be one explanation for why even popular TV shows reach only about one fifth of U.S. households, as even the "highly popular program ER never broke the 20% level, averaging ratings of 18%" (Sherry, 2002, pp. 207–208).

Newspaper Exposure

Groundbreaking science associated with human genetics has been headlined in newspapers for nearly a century (Condit, 1999). Newspapers have been found to have the highest impact regarding health campaign channels, contributing more to knowledge gains than television or print (Schooler, Chaffee, Flora, & Roser, 1998). In turn, knowledge has been found to be a necessary although not sufficient criteria in the formation of self-efficacy (Bandura, 1997). Newspaper stories about genetic testing emphasize doing good and avoiding harm (Craig, 2000) and also emphasize the role of personal behaviors and environments in addition to genes on health (Condit, 1999). This suggests that those who are exposed to newspaper stories about human genetics and health will have increased knowledge and improved perceptions of self-efficacy in the domain of genes and health. How RF may affect this process has not been examined. Newspaper reporters acknowledge that different religions take varied positions in the discussion of human genetics, but journalists "lack training in how to report on religions let alone how to decipher science jargon" (Valenti, 2002, p. 59). Research that examines newspaper reporting about religious content is limited to the religion section of daily papers (Valenti, 2002).

In sum, Figure 1 depicts a theoretical model derived from previous theory and research in the domains of religiosity, media use, and behavioral health outcomes. Self-efficacy is impacted by knowledge, response efficacy, and media exposure (Bandura, 1997). Response efficacy is linked to knowledge and media exposure (Bandura, 1997). In turn, knowledge depends on media exposure (Bandura, 1997). Based on a small but significant literature associating religiosity with media use, religiosity is depicted as impacting media exposure. The relation between religiosity and exposure to various modalities is uncertain, comprising one focus of this research. Moreover, the relations between different media and behavioral health outcomes associated with genes and health is speculative, leading to the following questions:

RQ2:   Does (1) intrinsic or (2) extrinsic religiosity relate to exposure to (a) movies, (b) daytime televised talk shows, (c) prime time medical and crime shows, or (d) newspapers with content about human genetics?

RQ3:   Does exposure to (1) movies, (2) daytime televised talk shows, (3) prime time medical and crime shows, or (4) newspapers with content about human genetics relate to (a) knowledge, (b) response efficacy, or (c) self-efficacy about genes and health?

METHOD

Participants and Procedures

Participants ($N = 858$) were recruited from four community-based geographic locations. To obtain an economically, racially, and educationally diverse sample, the geographic locations included two towns near large land grant universities, one in the southeast and one in the northeast, and two metropolitan cities, one in the southeast and one in the northeast. In the southeast, surveys were administered at a health fair, restaurants, churches, retailers, barbershops, beauty parlors, an airport, and laundromats, as well as the university ($n = 512$; 59.7%). In the northeast, data were collected at a train station, a bus station, an outlet mall, and a business office, as well as at a large, land grant university ($n = 292$; 34%). Some participants completed an online version of the survey ($n = 54$; 6.3%).

The sample included 339 men, 482 women, and 37 who did not report their gender. The self-identified ethnic and racial background of participants was primarily Black ($n = 273$; 32%) or White ($n = 470$; 55%), with the remaining participants reporting themselves as Asian ($n = 62$; 7%), Hispanic ($n = 23$; 3%), or Other ($n = 26$; 3%). Four participants did not report their racial background. The participants ranged in age from 18 to 73 years ($M = 29.59$; $SD = 10.42$). Education levels varied from less than high school (3%), high school diploma (15.7%), some college (23.8%), college degree (30.1%), vocational degree (3.7%), to advanced degrees (21.2%). The majority of participants with advanced degrees had not taken a genetics course in college (81.3%). Most participants (63%) did not have children, whereas 24.3% had one or two children and 11.8% had three or more children. When asked about overall religious attitude, 33.2% considered themselves to be very religious, about half (49%) reported being somewhat religious, 11.7% were not religious, and 5.6% were somewhat negative or very negative toward religion.

The survey that participants completed grew out of a larger research project associated with communicating genetics information to the lay public (Parrott, Silk, & Condit, 2003). Items were constructed through consultation with a lay advisory committee, an expert committee, a review of related literature, and formative research. The survey contained several scales of particular interest in this study including religiosity, self-efficacy, response efficacy, knowledge about genes, and exposure to information about genes and health through the media. Only these scales will be discussed and considered in the subsequent analyses. The descriptive statistics for survey items included in the following scales were examined, and all items were within the acceptable range for skewness and kurtosis of -2 to $+2$.

Religiosity. The scales for intrinsic and extrinsic religiosity came from Genia's (1993) revision of Allport and Ross' (1967) religiosity scale. Intrinsic religiosity was assessed using three items: (a) I try hard to carry my religion over into all my other dealings in life, (b) my religion is what lies behind my whole approach to life, and (c) religion answers many questions about the meaning of life ($M = 3.54$, $SD = 1.07$; $\alpha = .86$). Four items assessed extrinsic religiosity: (a) an important purpose of prayer is to get relief from my problems, (b) religion offers me comfort when misfortune strikes, (c) a primary purpose of prayer is to gain protection, and (d) an important purpose of prayer is to gain acceptance of misfortune ($M = 3.36$, $SD = .86$; $\alpha = .70$).

Self-Efficacy. Self-efficacy was assessed via use of three items: (a) I understand how to assess the role of genes for health, (b) I know how to assess my genetic risk for disease, and (c) I can explain genetic issues to people ($M = 2.52$; $SD = .80$; $\alpha = .71$).

Response efficacy. Response efficacy was assessed via four items: (a) genetics research can help women have healthier babies, (b) genetics research helps humans to live healthier lives, (c) genetics research helps humans to live longer, and (d) genetics research improves humans' quality of life. Reliability for the scale was acceptable ($M = 3.67$, $SD = .64$; $\alpha = .71$).

Genetic knowledge. Participants' knowledge about human genetics was measured using a five-item scale composed of the following statement: (a) every gene is able to mutate or change; (b) changes in your genes can be inherited; (c) changes in genes can occur over a lifetime; (d) every time a cell reproduces, there is a chance of error; and (e) changes in genes can be caused by chemicals. Participants responded by agreeing or disagreeing with each statement. Responses were dummy coded and summed together to form a scale ($M = 3.74$, $SD = 1.24$; $\alpha = .77$).

Media exposure. Four media scales were created to measure frequency of: exposure to movies with content about human genetics, exposure to daytime talk shows with content about human genetics, exposure to prime time medical and crime shows with content about human genetics, and exposure to newspaper articles related to human genetics research. The movie exposure scale was comprised of the following two questions: (a) I watch movies that show how the environment harms human genes, and (b) I watch movies that show how genes affect human health ($M = 1.98$, $SD = .86$; $\alpha = .79$). The talk show exposure scale was comprised of three questions including the following: (a) I see talk shows that discuss the effects of genes on human health, (b) I see talk shows that discuss how the environment harms human genes, and (c) I see talk shows that discuss how people's behaviors affect what their genes do ($M = 1.83$, $SD = .79$; $\alpha = .85$). The TV medical and crime show exposure scale contained two questions: (a) I watch medical drama shows on TV, and (b) I watch crime drama shows on TV ($M = 2.83$, $SD = 1.08$; $\alpha = .76$). The newspaper exposure scale contained two questions: (a) I read newspaper articles that discuss the effects of genes on human health, and (b) I read newspaper articles that discuss how the environment harms human genes ($M = 2.28$, $SD = .92$; $\alpha = .83$).

RESULTS

To answer the macroresearch questions associated with this research, bivariate correlations were computed (see Table 1). The results revealed significant correlations between extrinsic and intrinsic religiosity ($r = .53$, $p < .001$), self-efficacy and response efficacy ($r = .09$, $p < .001$), knowledge with self-efficacy ($r = .14$, $p < .001$), and response efficacy ($r = .09$, $p < .05$). Relations also existed between the media exposure variables and the religiosity, knowledge, and efficacy variables as summarized in Table 1. Structural equation modeling was used to assess the multiple linear relations, further examining the impact of RF on behavioral health outcomes with the theoretical model depicted in Figure 1 as a guide. Data were first entered into a database using the Statistical Package for the Social Sciences. Mean replacement was used, as nearly all surveys were complete, and for variables with missing values, less than 2% of the data were missing (Curran, West, & Finch, 1996). AMOS 4 was used to envision simultaneously the influence of intrinsic and extrinsic religiosity on exposure to media with genetic information and the behavioral health outcomes, and relations between media exposure to genetic information and knowledge, response efficacy, and self-efficacy.

TABLE 1
Bivariate Correlations Between Intrinsic Religiosity, Knowledge,
Self-Efficacy, Response Efficacy, and Media

	IR	ER	NP	TV	TS	MV	KN	SE	RE
Intrinsic Religiosity (IR)	1.0	.53**	−.12**	.04	.04	−.02	−.03	.03	.01
Extrinsic Religiosity (ER)		1.0	−.06	.05	.10**	.04	−.03	.04	.07*
Newspaper NP			1.0	.12**	.39**	.44**	.12**	.30**	.03
TV				1.0	.23**	.10**	.01*	.06	.11**
Talk Show (TS)					1.0	.51*	.08	.213*	.05
Movie (MV)						1.0	.11**	.27**	.09*
Knowledge (KN)							1.0	.14**	.09*
Self-Efficacy (SE)								1.0	.09*
Response Efficacy (RE)									1.0

*$p < .05$. **$p < .01$.

Test of the Overall Model

A covariance matrix was computed for use in developing a path diagram to visualize the set of proposed relations. The data fit the general theoretical relations depicted in Figure 1. The path diagram in Figure 2 illustrates the specific significant paths, such that knowledge did predict self-efficacy and response efficacy, media use impacted these behavioral outcomes, and religiosity did impact media use and the behavioral health outcomes. Several models using the total data set of 858 participants, as well as subsamples that included just European Americans ($n = 470$) and just African Americans ($n = 273$), were examined. The results for the total sample differed in terms of the strength of some relations retained in the final model, and the Tucker–Lewis index (TLI) and the comparative fit index (CFI) values when compared to the two subsamples. The path diagram in Figure 2 represents a model derived to visualize the most important relations overall, with all path coefficients significant at the $p < .05$ level. Only the results for the total sample are reported. The squared multiple correlations ranged from .015 for newspaper to .327 for movies; talk show = .165; TV = .053; knowledge = .015; response efficacy = .023; and self-efficacy = .125. The chi-square value was not significant ($\chi^2 (21) = 21.48; p = .43$). Several indicators were used to assess model fit. The TLI

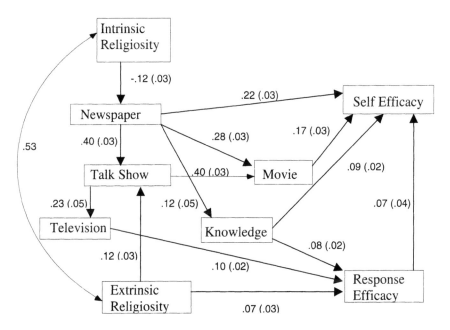

FIGURE 2   Religiosity's relation to media exposure and behavioral health outcomes. Model includes standardized estimates with associated standard errors in parentheses.

= .99, the CFI = 1.00, the Root Mean Square Error of Appproximation = .03, and the Standardized Root Mean Square Residual (SRMR) = .02. These values for CFI and SRMR have been found to reject reasonable proportions of misspecified models with sample sizes greater than 250 but less than 1,000 (Hu & Bentler, 1999). Next, the model is discussed in terms of the research questions.

RQ1. The first research question assessed the role of RF for the behavioral health outcomes of knowledge and self-efficacy and response efficacy. Intrinsic religiosity was not directly related to any of the behavioral health outcomes assessed in this research. Extrinsic religiosity had a significant association with response efficacy ($z = 2.00, p < .05$).

RQ2. The second research question assessed the role of RF in predicting use of media with genetic health content. Intrinsic and extrinsic religiosity were not directly related to exposure to movies with content about human genetics. A significant association between extrinsic religiosity and talk show exposure to information about genes and health was found ($z = 3.82, p < .001$), but no relation existed between intrinsic religiosity and talk shows. The model also revealed no significant relation between RF (intrinsic and extrinsic religiosity) and exposure to prime time medical and crime shows. Intrinsic religiosity was negatively associated with exposure to newspaper content about genes and health ($z = -3.59, p < .001$), but no significant relation existed between extrinsic religiosity and exposure to newspaper content related to genes and health.

RQ3. The third research question addressed the role of media exposure to behavioral health outcomes associated with genes and health. Exposure to movies with content about human genetics was associated with self-efficacy ($z = 4.64, p < .01$), but was not significantly associated with knowledge or response efficacy. Exposure to daytime televised talk shows with content about human genetics was not significantly associated with knowledge, self-efficacy, or response efficacy. Exposure to information about genes and health through talk shows was significantly associated with exposure to genetic information through movies ($z = 13.26, p < .001$) and television ($z = 6.89, p < .001$). Exposure to prime time medical and crime television shows was directly related to response efficacy ($z = 2.99, p < .01$). However, exposure to prime time medical and crime shows was not significantly related to self-efficacy or knowledge, or other media modalities. Exposure to newspaper articles about genes and health was associated with genetic knowledge ($z = 3.59, p < .05$) and self-efficacy ($z = 6.09, p < .001$). However, exposure to newspaper articles was not directly related to response efficacy. Information gained through newspapers was significantly associated with information gained through movies ($z = 9.15, p < .001$) and talk shows ($z = 12.64, p < .001$).

DISCUSSION

There is a tendency to pit science against religion in discourse associated with frontiers of discovery around human genetic research. The implicit assumption is that belief in God's role for humans denies belief in science and scientific explanations. Such simplistic conceptions have been challenged in the past, with the results of this research further supporting the need to envision the role of RF as a complex social and personal characteristic. RF was associated with media use and behavioral health outcomes related to human genetics, supporting the need for health communicators to attend to RF in the design of health promotion messages, "edu-tainment" interventions, and popular media assessments. The importance of this research in communicating about human genetics to lay audiences, directions for future research, ethical imperatives relating to both domains, as well as the limitations associated with this project, are considered.

Mapping of the human genome holds the promise of enhancing individual health and reducing the societal burden of disease. These outcomes are more likely as individuals gain knowledge about their own make-up together with the role of environments and personal behaviors on genetic expression. This study's results revealed that more knowledgeable participants were also more confident in their ability to impact the role of genes on health. Knowledge was also found to significantly impact perceptions of the efficacy of genetic technologies with response efficacy positively relating to self-efficacy as well. In an era of increasing reference to research relating genes to health, public understanding of the impact of environments and personal behavior as inputs affecting the role of genes is vital. Thus, efforts to understand the paths through which lay audiences gain confidence in their own control over genes and health become singularly critical.

At the broadest level, the findings support the conclusion that RF does not predetermine pessimistic attitudes about the role of genes in health, negatively impacting self-efficacy. Also, RF does not align with the belief that humans have overreached the boundaries of appropriateness for human intervention in genetics and health, negatively relating to response efficacy. In fact, the only direct relation found between RF and behavioral health outcomes was a positive one relating extrinsic religiosity to belief in the efficacy of genetic technologies. The impact of media on behavioral health outcomes associated with human genetics was revealing in its complexity, suggesting how lay audiences gain pathways to understanding. Exposure to movies with genetic content directly related to self-efficacy, perhaps highlighting the impact of dramatic portrayals contesting predetermined life courses (e.g., *Gattaca*). Newspaper use also positively directed the perceptions of individual control over genes and health, and actual knowledge about the role of genes for human health. Finally, exposure to TV crime and medical dramas related to enhanced perceptions of the efficacy of genetic technologies, whereas talk shows revealed no direct impact.

The results suggesting the impact of RF as a media gatekeeper offer important insights and directions for future research. Intrinsic religiosity was negatively related to newspaper use. Newspapers were an important source of both knowledge and self-efficacy, so individuals with more integrated RF have less exposure to this source and may be less knowledgeable and more deterministic in their views regarding genes and health, undesirable outcomes from a strategic health communication point of view. Newspaper use has been found to relate to positive evaluations of democratic institutions, including Congress, the court system, the presidency, public schools, and the news media, although a steady decline in readership has been observed over the past two decades (Moy & Pfau, 2000). Integrated patterns of religiosity may provide an explanation in both realms and suggest divergence in these two most critical elements of life in the United States—religion and politics.

Extrinsic religiosity was directly related to exposure to talk shows with genetic content. Although talk shows revealed no direct relation to behavioral health outcomes, exposure was an important predictor of both TV and movie use. To better understand how these modalities impact one another as sources of influence associated with human genetics, direct analysis of content from all three is needed, together with viewing patterns. Talk shows may provide the outlet for actors that appear on TV and in movies to talk about these outlets, influencing viewer consumption patterns. Alternatively, the explicit content of talk shows may have no bearing on motivating exposure to particular TV and movie content, but rather viewers of one of these media modalities may simply reveal a pattern of use that encompasses all three modalities.

Ethical Considerations

The findings that individuals with more integrated patterns of RF are less often exposed to human genetic content in newspapers, and that newspaper exposure directly impacts both self-efficacy and knowledge, suggests that this audience segment provides a niche that health communicators may target in efforts to impact illness causation frameworks. To do so, however, represents a targeting dilemma, so that health communicators need to assess carefully who needs to be reached with messages relating to human genetics (Guttman, 1997). If the desire is to reach all citizens with the intent of establishing a baseline of understanding in this realm, failure to apply the knowledge gained from this research represents a targeting dilemma based on ignoring the fact that current media are not reaching different audience segments equally.

Limitations

This research was limited in its geographic specificity, with participants belonging to two regions of the United States. A more representative sample would incorporate participants across the globe and from various faith doctrines. Also, this research relied on the use of religiosity measures that very broadly capture individual religious faiths and therefore provide only a general sense of the effects. Research is needed to more precisely operationalize individual approaches to human genetics as a result of RF. These statements might include the following: "I can influence the impact of my genes on my health through prayer," or "God uses human genes to reward good behavior on earth." More specific faith beliefs may have more direct impacts on behavioral outcomes associated with genes and health. Additional research is also required to assess media patterns associated with RF, including whether use is reactionary, reflects lifestyles associated with homes in which one parent stays at home to devote full-time to raising the children, or some other variable.

CONCLUSIONS

One broad challenge associated with reaching intended audiences with health information is that "many patterns in media selection are likely a reflection of the extent to which the viewer perceives the messages as useful in achieving goals, as informative, or as consistent with or confirming of attitudes or beliefs" (Oliver, 2002, p. 513). Information about genetics and health in media content may satisfy individual aims associated with being healthy if the information contributes to knowledge, including, for example, the mutability of genes. This knowledge may in turn promote understanding about the role of personal behavior on genetic expression, self-efficacy, or the role of genetic technologies in identifying genetic precursors of disease, response efficacy. These outcomes are more likely to occur if media content that contains information about genetics and health is accurate and accessible to all audiences, regardless of RF. That will require most likely, however, careful consideration of and attention to RF.

ACKNOWLEDGMENT

This research was supported by Grant No. R06/CCR417219 from the Centers for Disease Control and Prevention in Atlanta, GA.

REFERENCES

Abelman, R. (1987). Religious television uses and gratifications. *Journal of Broadcasting & Electronic Media, 31,* 293–307.

Abelman, R., & Hoover, S. M. (1990). *Religious television: Controversies and conclusions.* Norwood, NJ: Ablex.

Allport, G. W., & Ross, J. M. (1967). Personal religious orientation and prejudice. *Journal of Personality and Social Psychology, 5,* 432–443.

Ashing-Giwa, K. (1999). Health behavior change models and their socio-cultural relevance for breast cancer screening in African American women. *Women & Health, 28,* 53–71.

Bachtell, R. K., Wang, Y. M., Freeman, P., & Risinger, F. O. (1999). Alcohol drinking produces brain region-selective changes in expression of inducible transcription factors. *Brain Research, 847,* 157–165.

Bandura, A. (1997). *Self-efficacy: The exercise of control.* New York: Freeman.

Bernstein, C. (1994). Talk show nation. *New Perspectives Quarterly, 11,* 22–27.

Birmingham, E. (2000). Fearing the freak: How talk TV articulates women and class. *Journal of Popular Film and Television, 28,* 133–139.

Christensen, H., & Griffiths, K. M. (2000). The Internet and mental health literacy. *Australian & New Zealand Journal of Psychiatry, 34,* 975–979.

Clark, J. W., & Dawson, L. E. (1996). Personal religiousness and ethical judgements: An empirical analysis. *Journal of Business Ethics, 15,* 359–373.

Collins, F. S., & McKusick, V. A. (2001). Implications of the human genome project for medical science. *Journal of the American Medical Association, 285,* 540–544.

Condit, C. M. (1999). *The meanings of the gene: Public debates about human heredity.* Madison: The University of Wisconsin Press.

Craig, D. A. (2000). Ethical language and themes in news coverage of genetic testing. *Journalism & Mass Communication Quarterly, 77,* 160–174.

Curran, P. J., West, S. G., & Finch, J. F. (1996). The robustness of test statistics to nonnormality and specification error in confirmatory factor analysis. *Psychological Methods, 1,* 16–29.

Davis, S., & Mares, M. (2002). Effects of talk show viewing on adolescents. *Journal of Communication, 48,* 69–86.

Dossey, L. (1993). *Healing words: The power of prayer and the practice of medicine.* New York: HarperCollins.

Egbert, N., & Parrott, R. (2001). Self-efficacy and rural women's performance of breast and cervical cancer detection practices. *Journal of Health Communication, 6,* 219–234.

Gattaca. (1997). Retrieved March 30, 2003, from http://www.movieweb.com/movie/gattaca

Genia, V. (1993). A psychometric evaluation of the Allport–Ross I/E scales in a religiously heterogeneous sample. *Journal of the Scientific Study of Religion, 32,* 284–290.

Gerbner, G., Gross, L., Hoover, S., Morgan, M., & Signorielli, N. (1984). *Religion and television.* Philadelphia: University of Pennsylvania Press.

Grabe, M. E. (2002). Maintaining the moral order: A functional analysis of 'The Jerry Springer Show.' *Critical Studies in Mass Communication, 19,* 409–426.

Guttman, N. (1997). Ethical dilemmas in health campaigns. *Health Communication, 9,* 155–190.

Harter, L. M., & Japp, P. M. (2001). Technology as the representative anecdote in popular discourses. *Health Communication, 13,* 409–426.

Hu, L., & Bentler, P. M. (1999). Cutoff criteria for fit indexes in covariance structure analysis: Conventional criteria versus new alternatives. *Structural Equation Modeling, 6,* 1–55.

Isaac, S. (2001, February). *CSI: Crime scene investigation. Plugged in: Television Reviews.* Retrieved March 30, 2003, from http://www.family.org/pplace/pi/tv/a0014878.html

Jackson, C. (2000). Little, violent, White: The bad seed and the matter of children. *Journal of Popular Film and Television, 28,* 64–73.

Kerr, A., Cunningham-Burley, S., & Amos, A. (1998). Drawing the line: An analysis of lay people's discussions about the new genetics. *Public Understanding of Science, 7,* 113–133.

Khoury, M. J. (1996). From genes to public health: The application of genetic technology in disease prevention. *American Journal of Public Health, 86,* 1717–1722.

Kline, K. N. (2003). Popular media and health: Images, effects, and institutions. In T. L. Thompson, A. M. Dorsey, K. I. Miller, & R. Parrott (Eds.), *Handbook of health communication* (pp. 557–583). Mahwah, NJ: Lawrence Erlbaum Associates, Inc.

Koenig, H. G., & Larson, D. B. (1998). Use of hospital services, religious attendance, and religious affiliation. *Southern Medical Journal, 91,* 925–932.

Krause, N., & Tran, T. V. (1989). Stress and religious involvement among older Blacks. *Journal of Gerontology: Social Sciences, 44,* S4–S13.

Kundrat, A. L., & Nussbaum, J. F. (2003). The impact of invisible illness on identity and contextual age across the life span. *Health Communication, 15,* 331–347.

Levin, J. S., & Schiller, P. L. (1987). Is there a religious factor in health? *Journal of Religion and Health, 26,* 9–36.

Lusanne, C. (1999). Assessing the disconnect between Black and White television audiences: The race, class and gender politics of 'Married…With Children.' *Journal of Popular Film and Television, 27,* 12–20.

Miller, J. D. (1983). Scientific literacy: A conceptual and empirical review. *Daedalus, 112*(2), 29–48.

Moy, P., & Pfau, M. (2000). *With malice toward all? The media and public confidence in democratic institutions.* Westport, CT: Praeger.

Ogamdi, S. O. (1994). African American students' awareness of sickle cell disease. *Journal of American College Health, 42,* 234–236.

O'Keefe, G. J., Boyd, H., & Brown, M. R. (1998). Who learns preventive health care information from where: Cross-channel and repertoire comparisons. *Health Communication, 10,* 25–36.

Oliver, M. B. (2002). Individual differences in media effects. In J. Bryant & D. Zillmann (Eds.), *Media effects* (2nd ed., pp. 507–524). Mahwah, NJ: Lawrence Erlbaum Associates, Inc.

Pargament, K. I. (1998). Patterns of positive and negative religious coping with major life stressors. *Journal for the Scientific Study of Religion, 37,* 710–724.

Parrott, R. L., Silk, K., & Condit, C. (2003). Diversity in lay perceptions of the sources of human traits: Genes, environments, and personal behaviors. *Social Science & Medicine, 56,* 1099–1109.

Priest, P. (1995). *Public intimacies: Talk show participants and tell all TV.* Cresskill, NJ: Hampton.

Salmon, C., & Atkin, C. (2003). Using media campaigns for health promotion. In T. L. Thompson, A. M. Dorsey, K. I. Miller, & R. Parrott (Eds.), *Handbook of health communication* (pp. 449–473). Mahwah, NJ: Lawrence Erlbaum Associates, Inc.

Schooler, C., Chaffee, S. H., Flora, A., & Roser, C. (1998). Health campaign channels: Tradeoffs among reach, specificity, and impact. *Human Communication Research, 24,* 410–432.

Sherry, J. L. (2002). Media saturation and entertainment-education. *Communication Theory, 12,* 206–224.

Simpson, M. R., & King, M. G. (1999). "God brought all these churches together": Issues in developing religion-health partnerships in an Appalachian community. *Public Health Nursing, 16,* 41–49.

Smith, S. L., Nathanson, A. I., & Wilson, B. J. (2002). Prime-time television: Assessing violence during the most popular viewing hours. *Journal of Communication, 52*(1), 84–111.

Vanderford, M. (1999). Television and religious values: A case study of ER and moral ambiguity. In F. Eigo (Ed.), *Religious values at the threshold of the third millennium* (pp. 33–73). Villanova, PA: Villanova University Press.

Valenti, J. M. (2002). Communication challenges for science and religion. *Public Understanding of Science, 11,* 57–63.

Religious Identity and Smoking Behavior Among Adolescents: Evidence From Entering Students at the American University of Beirut

Rema Adel Afifi Soweid
Department of Health Behavior and Education
Faculty of Health Sciences, American University of Beirut

Marwan Khawaja
Department of Epidemiology and Population Health
Faculty of Health Sciences, American University of Beirut

Mylene Tewtel Salem
Center for Research on Population and Health
Faculty of Health Sciences, American University of Beirut

This survey investigation examines the association between religious identity and smoking behavior in a sample of older adolescents entering the university in Beirut, Lebanon. A culturally appropriate item of religiosity was developed for data collection. Results suggest that religious identity is inversely associated with regular smoking among male and female adolescents, after adjusting for sociodemographic, behavioral, personal, and environmental risk factors. The pattern of associations between weak religious identity, other risk factors, and smoking suggests that risk mechanisms may be gender-differentiated. Overall, findings suggest functional religiosity in late adolescence may assist in promoting the health and decreasing the morbidity of both men and women. Implications for future research are discussed.

Identity has traditionally been conceptualized to emanate from structural arrangements such as ethnicity, class, and gender. More recently, agency (personal perceptions of self identity) has been suggested to be assuming increasing importance

Requests for reprints should be sent to Rema Adel Afifi Soweid, Department of Health Behavior and Education, Faculty of Health Sciences, American University of Beirut, New York Office: 3 Dag Hammarskjold Plaza, 8th floor, New York, NY 10017. E-mail: ra15@aub.edu.lb over structure as a result of the contextual issues of late modernity (Denscombe, 2001). Adolescence is a time during which personal identities begin to form. In fact, the exploration of identity is socially sanctioned and encouraged during adolescence (Adams et al., 2001). Identity formation is considered to be a developmental process. Personal identity has been defined into four categories based on outcomes of crisis management: achieved (emerged from crisis with a clear commitment), moratorium (experiencing crisis but without clear commitment), foreclosed (committed to particular identity without experiencing crisis), and diffused (persons with no identity commitments, and no desire to explore such commitments). The latter two are considered to be the least developed.

More developed identity has been linked to more positive health outcomes (Hunsberger, Pratt, & Pancer, 2001). This article focuses on religiosity as a component of identity. Religion can play a part in the discovery of identity (Hunsberger et al., 2001), and religious identity (RI) is both social and personal, suggesting that messages from social networks may contribute to the formation and maintenance of RI. Focusing on RI as an indicator of personal and social identity can be justified in the context of Lebanon as both public and private spheres are to a great extent influenced by religion. In a political agreement after independence from the French mandate in 1943, the top positions in the Lebanese political bureaucracy were divided among Muslim and Christian sects (Joseph, 1997). The public endorsement of religion is also indicated through legal structures that are religiously framed. Thus, all family matters of birth, marriage, death, and inheritance are processed through a religious court rather than a secular one (Salibi, 1988). Religion has been able to permeate politics, because sectarian representation is legitimized by the state. This condition has obstructed a true national identity and the existence of a true national subject (Joseph, 1997). This public sphere of endorsement affects personal status codes and influences decisions at a very personal level. Personal identity cards list religious affiliation, and decisions on such personal matters as marriage are affected by the sectarian laws of the state.

The epidemiologic link between religion (religiosity) and positive health outcomes has been documented in several reviews (Chatters, 2000; Ellison & Levin 1998; Levin 1996). The central finding is that the protective effects of religion seem to transcend morbidity and mortality, as well as numerous physical and mental health outcomes. In addition, the positive effects of religiosity appear to be consistently robust, as many studies reviewed attempt to control for demographic characteristics (e.g., age, sex, socioeconomic background, race, and ethnicity) and other potential confounds. Progress in research on the relation between religiosity and health depends on further resolution of several important conceptual and measurement or methodological issues (Chatters, 2000). Egbert, Mickley, and Coeling (this issue), provide an in-depth review, but measures of religion reflecting variation in conceptual emphasis tend to divide into three different dimensions: (a) organizational and affiliation, (b) behavioral, and (c) subjective, or functional (Chatters, 2000; Ellison & Levin, 1998). The affiliation dimension, used extensively in early research on the religion–health connection (Strawbridge, Cohen, Shema, & Kaplan, 1997), classified persons according to membership in various religious denominations, and studies focused on those groups with beliefs and behaviors known to be health-promoting (e.g., Seventh-Day Adventists), and compared respective health outcomes between denominations. As scholarship in this area of research progressed, the organizational and affiliation measure was replaced by the behavioral dimension, which classifies persons according to religiosity (e.g., frequency of overtly religious behaviors, such as attendance at services, or prayers). As the multidimensionality of religion and religiosity became clearer, awareness of the need for concurrent measurement of the perceived (i.e., subjective or functional) dimension of religion in relation to health outcomes emerged. This functional dimension of religion incorporates attitudes, beliefs, values, experiences, and perceptions relevant to the meaning of religiosity to individuals (Chatters, 2000). Discussion of the function of religion in people's lives began in the 1960s conceptualized as intrinsic or extrinsic motivation toward religion (Allport & Ross, 1967). A third orientation, a quest orientation, relates to individuals' involvement in existential questioning and dialogue (Batson, Schoenrade, & Ventis, 1993).

Investigators have begun to focus on subpopulations such as adolescents, in an effort to produce a greater understanding of the relation between religion and health. Wallace and Forman (1998) included measures of each of the aforementioned dimensions (organization, behavioral, and functional) of religion to determine the influence of religiosity on adolescents' engagement in health risk behaviors. Using bivariate analyses, they found (with few exceptions) that each of the religiosity dimensions positively related to wearing seat belts, healthy dietary behavior, exercise, and appropriate sleep patterns. Conversely, the religiosity dimensions negatively related to carrying a weapon, interpersonal violence, riding or driving while intoxicated, and substance use or abuse. These findings have been supported by other research in the area of substance use and abuse (Atkins, Oman, Vesely, Aspy, & McLeroy, 2002; Pullen, Modrcin-Talbott, West, & Muenchen, 1999; Strote, Lee, & Wechsler, 2002; Sutherland & Shepherd, 2001; Whooley, Boyd, Gardin, & Williams, 2002), as well as studies which extended the protective relation of religiosity to sexual activity among young persons (Holder et al., 2000; Lammers, Ireland, Resnick, & Blum, 2000).

Research focused on factors influencing smoking among adolescents and young adults has also supported the salutary effect of religiosity (Atkins et al., 2002; Bell, Wechsler, & Johnston, 1997; Sutherland & Shepherd, 2001; Whooley et al., 2002). All three of these studies included the behavioral dimension, one (Whooley et al., 2002) included the affiliation dimension, and one (Sutherland & Shepherd, 2001) included the functional dimension of religion and religiosity. All of these investigations found an inverse correlation between behavioral religiosity and smoking, with adolescents and young adults who attended religious services more frequently being less likely to be cigarette smokers. In addition, during a 3-year follow-up period, nonsmokers who attended religious services more frequently were less likely to begin smoking cigarettes, and smokers who also attended services more frequently were more likely to quit smoking during the same follow-up period (Whooley et al., 2002). Finally, of various youth assets (protective factors) explored in these studies, religiosity was most effective against tobacco use, even after controlling for demographic factors. This research aims to increase knowledge related to functional religiosity and health behaviors of older adolescents (specifically smoking), and contributes to the literature by extending its scope to a country within the developing world, namely Lebanon. The research represents an exploratory test of the following hypothesis:

H1:   Fragmented or weak, RI among older adolescents contributes to smoking, independently of other established risk factors.

CONTEXT

Lebanon is a country in the Eastern Mediterranean region with a population of approximately 3.5 million (World Health Organization, 2003a). Lebanon has a very diverse racial and ethnic background. Political tensions have prevented the gathering of census data; the last national census in Lebanon was conducted in 1932. However, it is well known that Lebanon includes 18 religious denominations, and six major religious groups: Christians of Maronite, Greek Catholic, and Greek Orthodox faiths, and Muslims of Sunni, Shiite, and Druze faiths (Deeb, 1997). Smoking is quite common in Lebanon. Two forms of tobacco are most widely used: the cigarette and the water pipe. This research focuses only on cigarette smoking. There have been no national surveys of cigarette smoking in Lebanon, so prevalence statistics rely on results of community studies. These indicate prevalence rates for adults (19 years and older) that range from about 40% (MacKay & Eriksen, 2002) to 52.6% for current smoking and 67.2% for ever smoking (World Health Organization, 2003b).

Contrary to other countries in the region, rates of smoking among men and women are quite similar. About 46% of men smoke as compared to 35% of women (MacKay & Eriksen, 2002). As for youth smoking, approximately 11% of youth (15 to 18 years) are current smokers and 41% have ever tried smoking (World Health Organization, 2003b). Data from a select sample of entering university students (16 to 21 years) indicate that about 65% have ever tried smoking cigarettes, 34% had smoked on 1 or more days during the past 30 days, and 7% had smoked 11 or more cigarettes per day during the past month (Shediac-Rizkallah et al., 2000–2001). Rates for men and women did not differ significantly for ever smoking (67% and 63%, respectively) or for smoking 11 or more cigarettes per day during the last month (8.6% and 5.9%, respectively) but were significantly different for current smoking (39% and 28%, respectively). Cigarettes are widely available, as there is no age limit on the purchase of cigarettes and no ban on their advertisement. Cigarette prices range from L.L. 500 for the local brand to L.L. 2,000 for multinational brands (U.S. $1 = L.L. 1,500), making them affordable for all socioeconomic segments of the population.

METHOD

Instrument Development

In the fall of 1997, a group of faculty members of the American University of Beirut's (AUB) Faculty of Health Sciences initiated the Surveillance and Intervention for Behavioral Risk factors (SIBER) project. The project focused on university students, and as an initial activity, the group members designed a written survey to obtain data on a wide range of health risk behaviors (including, but not limited to, smoking) and offered the survey to all entering students at AUB. The survey and its methodology of administration were approved by the University Research Board as well as by the University's Board of Deans. The SIBER survey was developed as a result of an extensive search of the literature. SIBER working group members included professionals in the disciplines of epidemiology and biostatistics, health behavior and education, health services administration, environmental health, and family medicine. Many items were adapted from several previous studies, including the 1997 Centers for Disease Control and Prevention's Youth Risk Behavior Survey (Centers for Disease Control and Prevention, 2003). The survey is thus considered to have content validity.

The survey instrument includes 15 lifestyle and behavioral risk factors: general health status, health service utilization, health information sources, exercise, nutrition, disordered eating, oral hygiene, alcohol and drug use, tobacco use, sexual and reproductive health, unintentional injuries, intentional injuries, mental health, social support, and demographics. The survey was intentionally broad as it served as a starting point to the definition of priorities for intervention. To maximize response rate, surveys that cover many behaviors must be limited in scope and depth of understanding within each behavior. As a result, one-item measures were included and ultimately taken as preliminary indicators of prevalence of health risk behaviors. This may limit confidence in validity and reliability of measurement but is an important first step in identification of priorities. In-depth follow-up research focused on specific priorities must then be vigilant in instrumentation and measurement of psychometric properties. More extensive details about the survey, its development, methodology, and general findings can be found in Shediac-Rizkallah et al. (2000–2001).

Site, Participants, and Procedure

The AUB, situated in the capital of Lebanon, is a private coeducational university attended by approximately 5,000 students. The university serves as a regional leader in higher education and accommodates the cultural and religious diversity of the country and the Middle East. The survey was administered during a required (English) class for all entering students at AUB during the fall term of 1998. Over 3 consecutive days of administration, a total of 954 (90.1% of entering students— 9% did not take English in this semester) respondents completed the entire questionnaire. The refusal rate (0.9%) was very low.

Measurements

Selected items from the SIBER survey relevant to this study were abstracted for analysis. The items were selected based on a model that emphasizes sociodemographic, personal, behavioral, and environmental influences on smoking (Tyas & Pederson, 1998). Identity is not included in this model and was added to explore its contribution to tobacco use.

Index of religious identity. The primary predictor variable, RI, was conceptualized as consisting of two dimensions: strength of religiosity, as perceived by the respondent, and the functional impact of religiosity on daily activities. The questionnaire included two items that fairly captured these dimensions. The first item asked the following: To what extent do you consider yourself a religious person? The second item asked the following: To what extent do your religious beliefs affect the way you conduct your daily life? For answers to both items, a 4-point, Likert-type scale was used, ranging from *very much* to *not at all*. The two religiosity items were cross-classified and scores were combined into correspondingly meaningful weights, resulting in a trilevel index of RI. Respondents who indicated that the functional impact of religiosity was *very much/somewhat* and their perceived strength of religiosity was *very much/somewhat* were classified as one group with a score of 1, strong religious identity; those who indicated that the strength of religiosity was *very much/somewhat* but the functional impact was *little/not at all,* plus those who perceived the strength of their religiosity to be *little/not at all* but the functional impact to be *very much/somewhat,* were classified as one group with a score of 2, moderate religious identity; and those whose perceived strength of religiosity was *little/not at all* and the functional impact was *little/not at all* formed a third group that was scored as 3, weak religious identity. Thus, the Religiosity Index assessed the balance between respondents' perceived "religious feelings" and the functional impact of religiosity experienced in conducting daily life.

Control variables.   Only factors that had been shown by Tyas and Pederson (1998) to have a previous empirically significant association with the outcome variable were retained and used as control variables. This criterion produced the following control variables: (a) age of adolescent (16–17, 18, 19+), (b) availability of pocket money (none, 1–50, >50–100, >100 in thousand Lebanese Lira per week where 1, 500 L.L. = U.S. $1), (c) nationality (Lebanese, Lebanese and other, and non-Lebanese), (d) residing outside Lebanon for at least 1 year (yes, no), (e) peer smoking (none/a few, most/all), (f) household member smoking (never to sometimes, frequently), (g) satisfaction with academic work (often, sometimes/never), (h) alcohol use last month (0 day, 1+ days), (i) physical fight past 12 months (0 times, 1+ times), (j) regular exercise defined as any physical activity performed 3 times a week for at least 20 min each (yes, no), (k) physical or mental health problem negatively impacting the conduct of usual activities within the past 30 days (0 days, 1+ days), (l) use of sedatives to relax (never, rarely/often), (m) use of one or more mind–body relaxation techniques (never, sometimes, often), (n) occurrence of tension, migraine, or headache (never/rarely/sometimes, often), (o) perceived control over health (a great deal, some, no), and (p) and family and friends social support (high, medium, low).

Level of social support was measured using a battery of five questions encompassing perception of actual and potential support from family and friends. Each respondent was asked the following: "If you have a problem, how often is it that you can count on your family or relatives (friends) for: (1) helping with your daily tasks, (2) connecting you to people that can help, (3) emotional support, (4) financial support, (5) providing you with helpful information?" These questions tap three types of social support: emotional (3), instrumental (1, 2, 4), and informational (2, 5; Heaney & Israel, 2002). For each item, four answers were possible: *always, often, sometimes,* and *never.* Social support indexes were created by summing the scores and dividing the frequencies into three approximately equal groupings of high, medium, and low social support.

Smoking.   The outcome (dependent) variable was regular smoking behavior. The instrument included various commonly used measures of smoking behavior, including number of cigarettes smoked per day, number of days smoked during the last month, and self-perception of regular smoking. Regular smoking was measured by a direct question: "Do you consider yourself a regular smoker?" Those who answered yes (13.3%) were considered regular smokers. This item is a valid measure of regular smoking, as about 96% of self-reported regular smokers smoked 10 or more cigarettes per day during the last month. Similarly, about 96% of those who self-classified as "not regular smokers" smoked less than 10 cigarettes per day in the last month. Because measurement of RI was based on items indicating perceptions of respondents rather than objective measurements, the dependent variable was chosen to indicate subjective perceptions of extent of smoking. This decision was supported by similar results of the same analysis using other indicators of tobacco use (e.g., cigarettes smoked per day).

Analysis Approach

Prevalence of regular smoking by male and female adolescents was computed using a question about self-perceived smoking. Descriptive statistics were examined for associations between adolescents' RI, control variables, and smoking. Separate descriptive statistics were also examined for males and females. Multiple logistic regression was used to model the probability of regular smoking as a function of RI controlling for other relevant factors. Estimated regression coefficients from the fitted model were used to compute the adjusted odds ratios and 95% confidence interval to assess associations between RI and regular smoking, controlling for several risk, and protective factors.

RESULTS

The final sample for analysis included 954 students. Fifty-three percent of respondents were male, and 47% were female. Nineteen percent were ages 16 to 17, 64% were 18 years of age, and 17% were over 18 years old. Fifty-nine percent had lived outside Lebanon for at least a year. In addition, 66% were Lebanese only, 23% had dual nationalities including Lebanese, and 11% were non-Lebanese. With respect to pocket money received per week, 5% stated they received none, 42% received L.L. 50,000 or less, 35% received between L.L. 51,000 and L.L. 100,000, and 18% received more than L.L. 100,000. Distribution of the sample population on the Religiosity Index with scores 1 (*strong*) to 3 (*weak*) were, respectively, 48.8%, 20.2%, and 31.0%. Women had a stronger RI than men; the corresponding index scores were 55.3%, 19%, and 25.8% for women, and 42.9%, 21.2%, and 35.9% for men. There was no significant difference on the index by the status risk factors of age, nationality, pocket money, or living outside Lebanon.

As expected, regular smoking was strongly and consistently associated with religiosity: About 7% of students with strong RI were regular smokers, compared to over 23% of those reporting weak religiosity. Regular smoking was also positively associated with age, (having) pocket money, nationality and residence outside Lebanon, exposure to peer and household smoking, satisfaction with academic performance, alcohol use, no regular exercise, violent behavior, stress, control over health, negative health status, and family and friends' support (data not shown). To determine the net impact of religiosity on regular smoking, a logistic regression of regular smoking on all factors was conducted (see Table 1). Weak RI remained strongly associated with regular smoking, adjusting for all other factors (odds ratio of 3.40, $p < .001$). Other variables with strong and consistent associations with regular smoking were age, nationality, peer smoking, alcohol use, physical fights, no regular exercise, poor health impacting activities, any use of sedatives to relax, mind–body relaxation, and low level of friends' social support. No statistically significant associations were found in the full logistic regression model between regular smoking and availability of pocket money, lack of satisfaction with academic performance, perceived lack of control over one's health, or family social support.

Table 1 also reports results for men and women. Weak RI was strongly associated with smoking both for older adolescent males and females (odds ratio of 4.23, $p < .003$, and 3.95, $p<0.024$, respectively), regardless of the effects of other factors. Remarkably, only three other predictor variables show similar patterns of significant association for men and women: peer smoking and the two behavioral risk factors of alcohol use and physical fights. The remaining variables showed sex-specific patterns of association or none at all. Only one indicator of stress (the use of sedatives to relax) was a significant predictor of smoking among men. Conversely, age, nationality, perceived control over health, and social support variables were statistically significant for women, but not for men. In sum, sociodemographic and social support factors were specific predictors of female smoking, whereas behavioral and some personal factors were specific predictors for male smoking.

DISCUSSION

The primary finding of this study is that religiosity (measured by the RI as a functional dimension) was inversely associated with regular smoking among a sample of older adolescents. Put another way, the data supports the study hypothesis that fragmented or weak RI among older adolescents contributes to smoking. This primary association is independent of the effects of commonly known behavioral, personal, sociodemographic, and environmental risk factors for smoking, and is gender invariant. Thus, religiosity is empirically supported by this research as a protective factor against smoking over and above other identified factors, consistent with the previous literature concerning the general health effects of religiosity. RI should thus be added to explanatory models of smoking behavior.

Interestingly, no statistical differences were found in smoking among those with strong versus moderate RI overall or by gender. The significant differences were between those with strong as compared to weak RI. Although it seems reasonable to equate those with strong RI to persons with intrinsic motivation (Allport & Ross, 1967), it may be that those with moderate RI, as defined in this study, are not extrinsically oriented, but rather more similar to those with a quest orientation

TABLE 1
Logistic Regression: Religiosity and Regular Smoking Perception, With Controls

Independent Variables	Overall		Males		Females	
	Odds Ratio	p	Odds Ratio	p	Odds Ratio	p
Religiosity						
Strong	1.00		1.00		1.00	
Moderate	1.47	0.310	1.12	0.839	1.51	0.542
Weak	3.44	0.000	4.23	0.003	3.95	0.024
Sociodemographic						
Age						
16 to 17	1.00		1.00		1.00	
18	1.69	0.201	0.47	0.192	8.02	0.003
19+	4.01	0.003	1.63	0.410	19.3	0.002
Pocket money						
None	1.00		1.00		1.00	
Yes, ≤50,000	0.52	0.308	0.54	0.521	0.37	0.396
Yes, 50,001 to 100,000	1.43	0.570	1.59	0.633	1.64	0.695
Yes, >100,000	1.00	0.998	1.45	0.705	0.80	0.853
Nationality						
Lebanese only	1.00		1.00		1.00	
Lebanese and another	2.64	0.003	1.99	0.132	5.55	0.007
Non-Lebanese	2.35	0.034	1.51	0.498	8.87	0.002
Lived outside Lebanon						
No	1.00		1.00		1.00	
Yes	1.13	0.720	0.78	0.585	2.04	0.291
Environmental						
Peer smoking						
None—a few of them	1.00		1.00		1.00	
Most—all of them	7.21	0.000	7.27	0.000	17.40	0.000
Household smokers						
Never to sometimes	1.00		1.00		1.00	
Frequently to always	1.19	0.521	1.28	0.520	1.16	0.769
Behavioral						
Satisfying academic work						
Often	1.00		1.00		1.00	
Sometimes, rarely, never	1.27	0.474	1.20	0.705	0.69	0.544
Alcohol use						
0 days	1.00		1.00		1.00	
1 day or more	3.52	0.000	4.06	0.005	2.89	0.040
Physical fights						
Past 12 months						
0 time	1.00		1.00		1.00	
1 or more time	2.88	0.000	4.72	0.000	3.94	0.040
Regular exercise						
Yes	1.00		1.00		1.00	
No	2.05	0.012	2.08	0.063	2.44	0.110

(continued)

56

TABLE 1 *(Continued)*

Independent Variables	Overall		Males		Females	
	Odds Ratio	P	Odds Ratio	P	Odds Ratio	P
Personal						
Poor health impacts activities						
0 days	1.00		1.00		1.00	
1 or more days	1.76	0.045	1.32	0.474	2.90	0.055
Use sedatives to relax						
Never	1.00		1.00		1.00	
Rarely to often	2.49	0.018	5.19	0.003	1.57	0.543
Mind/body relaxation						
Often	1.00		1.00		1.00	
Sometimes/rarely	1.47	0.331	1.15	0.779	1.11	0.906
Never	3.60	0.005	3.02	0.080	3.95	0.169
Tension or migraine headaches						
Never, rarely, sometimes	1.00		1.00		1.00	
Often	1.46	0.268	1.45	0.493	1.24	0.705
Control over health						
No or little control	1.00		1.00		1.00	
Some control	0.83	0.594	1.65	0.351	0.32	0.067
A great deal of control	0.74	0.455	1.94	0.268	0.17	0.019
Social support from family						
High	1.00		1.00		1.00	
Medium	0.80	0.513	0.61	0.316	1.18	0.794
Low	1.74	0.117	0.70	0.503	5.58	0.006
Social support from friend						
High	1.00		1.00		1.00	
Medium	0.61	0.116	1.17	0.734	0.35	0.074
Low	0.22	0.000	0.38	0.090	0.11	0.011

(Genia, 1996). They would thus be searching for answers and therefore not consider themselves very religious but consider that religion did influence their lives, or consider themselves religious but not currently be practicing their religion in their daily life. The link between the measure of RI used in the current research and the functional orientation needs further investigation. This investigative research may be more qualitative in methodology to understand the characteristics of those individuals who classify themselves as having a moderate RI according to their answers to question items measuring intrinsic, extrinsic, and quest orientations.

Consistent with previous findings (Tyas & Pederson 1998), regular smoking among respondents was also associated with other classes of risk factors. These risk factors consist of sociodemographic (status) variables, such as age, pocket money, nationality and residence outside Lebanon; environmental variables such as exposure to peer and household smoking; behavioral variables, such as alcohol use, exercise, and violent behavior; and personal variables, such as stress, control over health, physical health status, and social support from family and friends. Salient gender differences also emerged. For male adolescents, RI influences smoking along with mostly behavioral factors, whereas for females, it does so with mostly personal and social support variables. Reviews of the religion–health connection (Chatters, 2000, Ellison & Levin, 1998) have identified several explanatory mechanisms for the relation between religiosity and health. These include, among others, the following: (a) religion regulating health behavior; (b) participating in services or as a member of a religious group providing expanded and denser social networks which has a direct and indirect effect on health (Heaney & Israel, 2002); (c) religion promoting positive attitudes, beliefs, and emotions which may promote health; and (d) religious attitudes and cognitions that provide effective coping resources for daily life stresses, and thus buffer the effect of stress on health. Our results may suggest that the religion–health connection in men is explained by the first pathway listed earlier—religion tends to regulate health behavior, whereas that of women is explained through the second pathway—the mediating effect of social networks, including religious social networks.

Limitations

The findings of this research must be interpreted with caution. Smoking status was assessed using only one item. Although this is not an uncommon practice in research on the association between tobacco use and religiosity (Atkins et al. 2002; Sutherland & Shepherd, 2001), the validity of one-item measures could be questionable. The specific measure used was chosen because it was a participant-perceived smoking status and thus has emic validity. It was felt to be appropriate as the counterpart to a participant-perceived measure of religiosity. Also, as mentioned earlier, analysis using other indicators of smoking yielded remarkably similar results.

The survey was cross-sectional. The use of a cross-sectional survey design necessitates that any conclusions about directions of causality are tentative. Also, the data were obtained from self-report. All reasonable means were used to maximize the validity of responses (e.g., ensuring anonymity and confidentiality); the usual limitations of self-report, such as social desirability and problems of recall, are applicable to data obtained from the RI.

There are also limits concerning the sample used in this study. That is, further research on religiosity and regular smoking should be conducted with cohorts of university students at all levels (sophomore, junior, senior, graduate), and including all universities in the country, before results can be generalized. In addition, AUB is a private university with one of the highest tuitions in the Middle East. Accordingly, AUB students as a whole do not reflect the full range of socioeconomic status within Lebanon (which contributes the majority of AUB alumni) or other countries in the region. Furthermore, every year a sizeable percentage of Lebanese youth does not choose to pursue higher education. Education level is a potential correlate of knowledge concerning the health risks of smoking. Thus, to produce generalizable associations and potential pathways in this research domain, the full spectrum of older adolescents' educational backgrounds should be represented in future studies.

Finally, the Middle East as a region is steeped in a particular religious history and a correspondingly unique identity. Whether the local population of concern is older adolescents, or any other Middle Eastern group, the perceived relevance of religion to daily life and therefore its functional impact may be different in this region compared to other regions of the world. Therefore, similar studies need to be conducted in other countries and regions of the world.

Ethical Issues

The central purpose of research and intervention conducted by public health and communication professionals involving religiosity is the application of science to an increased understanding of the processes through which religion has an influence on health. Results gained from such research cannot be used to value one type of person over another, or to discriminate against any persons—as this violates the universal declaration of human rights (United Nations, 2003) and public health code of ethics (Thomas, Sage, Dillenberg, & Guillory, 2002).

Another significant ethical concern focuses on the use of data favoring religiosity in health to try to preach a particular religious point of view, and to influence— and at the extreme, coerce, persons to take up religion. Although this is indeed a potential negative use of research involving religiosity, the identified impact of religion on health necessitates that we do not ignore it out of fear, but continue to explore and increase understanding of the exact processes of influence, while insuring the appropriate use of resulting information.

Problems related to ethical issues can be greatly limited by applying a participatory approach to all research and intervention involving dimensions of religiosity. A participatory approach includes members of the concerned population in all aspects of research and intervention planning, implementation, and evaluation. These members are thus influencing all decision making related to research and intervention.

Implications for Health Communication Researchers and Practitioners

Several implications for public health and health communication researchers and practitioners can be drawn from the results described in this article. RI is a critical variable in influencing the initiation of health risk behaviors, specifically smoking. Potentially, it could serve as a marker for risk and could be used, along with other variables, in the identification of target groups for intervention programs related to smoking prevention or control. Health communication messages could also benefit from the results. Many persons are not aware of the teachings of religion on smoking or other risk behaviors. Health communicators may point out the position of religion on smoking. This may result in an imbalance that the individual will act to decrease by changing his or her opinion about religion or by changing his or her opinion (and ultimately behavior) about smoking. The choice is more likely to be toward a change related to smoking, as religion is an integral part of self-concept and identity and thus harder to change. This communication related to the position religion has toward smoking or other risk behaviors can be communicated in the context of the family, the health professional relationship, through health communication mass media interventions, or through religious leaders. An evaluation of the influence of religious leaders on smoking rates indicated that the percentage of persons who stopped smoking in the village of an Abbot who discourages smoking was higher than that of a neighboring village. In addition, persons in the Abbot's villages were more likely to cite him as an important reason for stopping than health workers or family members (Religious Leaders and Health Promotion, 1993).

CONCLUSIONS AND FUTURE RESEARCH

RI protected older adolescents from smoking over and above the influence of known sociodemographic, personal, behavioral, and environmental factors. Further research is needed to replicate these results and extend them to other measures of tobacco use, and to other risk behaviors. In addition, research should identify the associations of the RI item with the functional dimensions of religion (Allport & Ross, 1967; Genia, 1996), other behavioral measures of religiosity, and the potential pathways of influence. The finding that religion joins behavioral variables to influence smoking in men, and personal and social variables to influence smoking in women, should motivate further, explanatory investigations of the meaning of religiosity for female and male older adolescents, thus contributing to elucidation of the causal pathways and mechanisms linking religion to health. As such, this study adds to the empirical substance of the literature, and also stimulates theoretical development. As suggested earlier, numerous opportunities exist to examine strategies to communicate religious views to adolescent audiences and their impact on attitudes and behavior.

ACKNOWLEDGMENT

We thank Dr. Walid Afifi for his invaluable contribution to the assessment of the health communication implications of the results. We also thank Mr. Kirk Hooks for editorial work on various versions of this manuscript.

REFERENCES

Adams, G. R., Munro, B., Doherty-Poirer, M., Munro, G., Petersen, A. R., & Edwards, J. (2001). Diffuse-avoidance, normative, and informational identity styles: Using identity theory to predict maladjustment. *Identity: An International Journal of Theory and Research, 1,* 307–320.

Allport, G. W., & Ross, M. (1967). Personal religious orientation and prejudice. *Journal of Personality and Social Psychology, 5,* 432–443.

Atkins, L. A., Oman, R. F., Vesely, S. K., Aspy, C. B., & McLeroy, K. (2002). Adolescent tobacco use: The protective effects of developmental assets. *American Journal of Health Promotion, 16,* 198–205.

Batson, C. D., Schoenrade, P., & Ventis, W. L. (1993). Dimensions of individual religion. In C. D. Batson, P. Schoenrade, & W. L. Ventis (Eds.), *Religion and the individual: A social–psychological perspective* (pp. 155–172). New York: Oxford University Press.

Bell, R., Wechsler, H., & Johnston, L. D. (1997). Correlates of college student marijuana use: Results of a US National survey. *Addiction, 92,* 571–581.

Centers for Disease Control and Prevention. (2003). *Youth risk behavior surveillance system.* Retrieved March 23, 2003, from http://www.cdc.gov/nccdphp/dash/yrbs/about_yrbss.htm

Chatters, L. M. (2000). Religion and health: Public health research and practice. *Annual Review of Public Health, 21,* 335–367.

Deeb, M. E. (1997). Introduction. In M. E. Deeb (Ed.), *Beirut: A health profile 1984–1994* (pp. 1–8). Beirut, Lebanon: American University of Beirut.

Denscombe, M. (2001). Uncertain identities and health-risking behaviour: The case of young people and smoking in late modernity. *British Journal of Sociology, 52,* 157–177.

Ellison, C .G., & Levin, J. S (1998). The religious–health connection: Evidence, theory and future directions. *Health Education and Behavior, 25,* 700–720.

Genia, V. (1996). I, E, quest, and fundamentalism as predictors of psychological and spiritual well-being. *Journal for the Scientific Study of Religion, 35,* 56–64.

Heaney, C. A., & Israel, B. A. (2002). Social networks and social support. In K. Glanz, B. K. Rimer, & F. Marcus Lewis (Eds.), *Health behavior and health education: Theory, research, and practice* (pp. 185–209). San Francisco: Jossey–Bass.

Holder, D. W., Durant, R. H., Harris, T. L., Henderson Daniel , J., Obeidallah, D., & Goodman, E. (2000). The association between adolescent spirituality and voluntary sexual activity. *Journal of Adolescent Health, 26,* 295–302.

Hunsberger, B., Pratt, M., & Pancer, S. M. (2001). Adolescent identity formation: Religious exploration and commitment. *Identity: An International Journal of Theory and Research, 1,* 365–386.

Joseph, S. (1997). The public/private—The imagined boundary in the imagined nation/state/community: the Lebanese case. *Feminist Review, 57,* 73–92.

Lammers, C., Ireland M., Resnick, M., & Blum, R. (2000). Influences on adolescents' decision to postpone onset of sexual intercourse: A survival analysis of virginity among youths aged 13 to 18 years. *Journal of Adolescent Health, 26,* 42–48.

Levin, J. S. (1996). How religion influences morbidity and health: Reflections on natural history, salutogenesis and host resistance. *Social Science and Medicine, 43,* 849–864.

MacKay, J., & Eriksen, M. (2002). *The tobacco atlas* (pp. 98–101). Geneva, Switzerland: World Health Organization.

Pullen, L., Modrcin-Talbott, M. A., West, W. R., & Muenchen, R. (1999). Spiritual high vs high on spirits: Is religiosity related to adolescent alcohol and drug abuse? *Journal of Psychiatric and Mental Health Nursing, 6,* 3–8.

Religious leaders and health promotion. (1993). *The Lancet, 341,* 1655.

Salibi, K. (1988), *A house of many mansions: The history of Lebanon reconsidered.* Berkeley: University of California Press.

Shediac-Rizkallah, M. C., Afifi-Soweid, R. A., Farhat, T., Yeretzian, J., Nuwayhid, I., Sibai, A., et al. (2000–2001). Adolescent health-related behaviors in postwar Lebanon: Findings among students at the American University of Beirut. *International Quarterly of Community Health Education, 20,* 115–131.

Strawbridge, W. J., Cohen, R. D., Shema, S. J., & Kaplan, G. A. (1997). Frequent attendance at religious services and mortality over 28 years. *American Journal of Public Health, 87,* 957–961.

Strote, J., Lee, J. E., & Wechsler, H. (2002). Increasing MDMA use among college students: Results of a national survey. *Journal of Adolescent Health, 30,* 64–72.

Sutherland, I., & Shepherd J. P. (2001). Social dimensions of adolescent substance use. *Addiction, 96,* 445–458.

Thomas, J. C., Sage, M., Dillenberg, J., & Guillory, V. J. (2002). A code of ethics for Public Health. *American Journal of Public Health, 92,* 1057–1059.

Tyas, S. L., & Pederson, L. L. (1998). Psychosocial factors related to adolescent smoking: A critical review of the literature. *Tobacco Control, 7,* 409–420.

United Nations, Office of the High Commissioner for Human Rights. (1948). *The Universal Declaration of Human Rights.* Retrieved March 24, 2003, from http://193.194.138.190/udhr/index.htm

Wallace, J. M., & Forman, T. A. (1998). Religion's role in promoting health and reducing risk among American youth. *Health Education and Behavior, 25,* 721–741.

Whooley, M. A., Boyd, A. L., Gardin, J. M., & Williams, D. R. (2002). Religious involvement and cigarette smoking in young adults: The CARDIA study. *Archives of Internal Medicine, 162,* 1604–1610.

World Health Organization. (2003a). *Lebanon.* Retrieved March 23, 2003, from http://www.who.int/country/lbn/en/

World Health Organization. (2003b). *Lebanon.* Retrieved March 23, 2003, from http://ww5.who.int/tobacco

HEALTH COMMUNICATION, *16*(1), 63–85

Grounding Research and Medical Education About Religion in Actual Physician–Patient Interaction: Church Attendance, Social Support, and Older Adults

Jeffrey D. Robinson and Jon F. Nussbaum
Department of Communication Arts & Sciences
The Pennsylvania State University

This article reviews the relation between social support and elder health, the so-cial-support dimensions of religion, the relation between church attendance and elder health, the place of religion in the biopsychosocial model of medicine, and medical education's position on physician–patient communication about religion. It then ex-amines the emergence of the topic of religion in actual visits. Data are 71 videotaped and transcribed, chronic-routine visits between 12 internal medicine physicians and their older patients. Religion was raised as a topic in 9 visits (13%). In every case, the topic was initiated by patients. The most frequent topic was church attendance (7 of 9 topics), which patients typically used as a contextualizing framework to relate and describe somatic problems. In no cases did physicians make efforts to support or fa-cilitate patients' church attendance, as is advocated by medical education. Implica-tions for medical education and the biopsychosocial model are discussed.

Roter (2000) identified the need for communication scholars to confront emerg-ing ethical issues in medicine, such as decision making in end-of-life discus-sions. Although not as publicly visible as cloning and stem cell research, an equally controversial issue is religion (Mills, 2002). There is no scientific evi-dence that functional and organic disease can be healed by the solicitation of di-vine power alone (Levin, 1996). However, there is evidence that religious beliefs

Requests for reprints should be sent to Jeffrey D. Robinson, Department of Communication Arts & Sciences, 234 Sparks Building, University Park, PA 16802-5201. E-mail: jdr12@psu.edu and behaviors are multifaceted health-protective factors, especially for older adults (Koenig, McCullough, & Larson, 2000). For medical educators and physicians, who have taken an oath to heal the sick, this presents a professional–ethical dilemma between prescribing behaviors and prescribing religion. It presents a similar dilemma for health care policymakers, who might consider, for example, granting frequent church attendees special health insurance rates (Koenig & Larson, 1998).

This article focuses on how religion—in particular, church attendance—emerges as a topic of discussion in visits where older adult patients are seeing internal medicine physicians for the purpose of dealing with chronic-routine problems. Regarding older adults, this article begins by briefly reviewing the relation between social support and health, how religion is a unique form of social support, and the relation between religion and health, with a focus on church attendance. It proceeds to review the place of religion in the biopsychosocial model of medicine and medical education's position on physician–patient communication about religion. Finally, it grounds research and medical education about religion in actual physician–patient communication by analyzing the frequency, content, and process of discussing religious topics.

OLDER ADULTS AND SOCIAL SUPPORT

A complex relation exists among physical and mental health, social support, and aging. A general myth associated with the aging process is that, as persons grow older, they can expect a steady decline in both social activity and health. Although it is true that older adults suffer from more chronic or long-term illnesses than younger adults, and although older adults visit their physicians and utilize health care systems more frequently than younger adults (Beisecker & Thompson, 1995), it is nevertheless the case that each successive cohort of older adults maintains an active lifestyle and a positive health profile throughout the great majority of their lives (Nussbaum, Pecchioni, Robinson, & Thompson, 2000). Active and healthy aging can be attributed to various advances in medicine, technology, and public health policy. However, communication scholars have been searching for the social–interactional correlates and causes of activity and good health throughout the aging process.

Numerous researchers have concluded that active participation within a social network of family and friends, together with positive perceptions toward social interaction, are key determinants of successful aging (Baltes & Baltes, 1990). Krause (2001) highlighted the work of Barrera (1986) in an attempt to understand why older adults who are embedded within supportive social networks not only enjoy better physical and mental health, but also significantly increase their odds of having a longer life. Barrera advanced three dimensions of social support that appear to be related to good health as persons age: (a) social embeddedness (i.e., frequency of contact with others), (b) received support (i.e., the amount of help actually provided by others), and (c) perceived support (i.e., satisfaction with received support). Norris and Kaniasty (1996) found that positive feelings of perceived support is the most predictive characteristic of social support on health and well-being in later life. House, Landis, and Umberson (1988) reviewed a quarter century of research linking social support to health and concluded that individuals who are socially isolated, and who have not constructed a reasonably strong social network of supportive relationships, are more likely to be physically and psychologically less healthy and are more likely to die at a younger age. Levin (2001), a social epidemiologist, went so far as to conclude that a lack of social support is a fundamental cause of disease.

RELIGION AS A UNIQUE FORM OF SOCIAL SUPPORT FOR OLDER ADULTS

Sociologists (e.g., Durkheim, 1951) and psychologists (e.g., James, 1978) have long theorized that religious beliefs and practices involve social and psychological mechanisms that are associated with health and well-being (Levin, 1996; Vanderpool & Levin, 1990). Religious events (e.g., weekly mass, prayer groups, Bible school, church-related social functions, etc.) offer preexisting reservoirs of individuals and activities that constitute, and facilitate the maintenance of, social support networks (Krause, 2001). For example, other congregants can provide a sense of belonging, fellowship, and cohesiveness, as well as provide instrumental and emotional resources, such as monitoring others for illness and providing encouragement, hope, and aid (Koenig & Larson, 1998).

Older adults can have a particularly difficult time maintaining connections to social-support networks, and thus have the potential to rate low on social embeddedness, received support, and perceived support. Without endorsing the decrement model of aging, the aging process is associated with socially isolating changes in persons' language skills, cognitive abilities, and competencies regarding relationships and communication (Nussbaum, Barringer, & Kundrat, 2002). As persons age, these factors, together with a host of others—such as the death of friends and family members, lessened mobility, stagnant finances, and forced relocation—can negatively affect the quantity and quality of social networks and support. For older adults, religion can be a unique source of social support. That is, as opposed to numerous social-support networks that are temporary across the life course (e.g., college associations, employment-related events, etc.), friend networks that shrink over the life course (e.g., due to relocation, friends' deaths, etc.), and family networks that shrink when older adults are relocated, one enduring, social-support network is organized religion.

Older (vs. younger) adults are more likely to experience mobility limitations that are obstacles to maintaining active social lives (e.g., inability to walk or drive). However, unlike many other social support networks, religious organizations typically facilitate transportation to and from events. Philosophically, religion tends to encourage social-support-related behaviors, such as staying married (Levin, 1996). Theologically, religions offer coping strategies that secular institutions do not, such as providing a sense of control over one's own actions (e.g., through prayer and ways of living), contextualizing stressful events in larger systems of meaning (e.g., fear of death), and ultimately turning over stressful events to a benevolent and concerned Other (e.g., God; Vanderpool & Levin, 1990). These latter aspects of "secondary control" are particularly helpful for older adults who, as a result, can spend more energy on positively interacting with others instead of negatively dwelling on their difficulties (Krause, Morgan, Chatters, & Meltzer, 2000).

Compared to middle-aged and younger adults, older adults are more likely to belong to formal religious organizations, pray, and attend church (McFadden, 1995). Unlike young and middle-aged adults, religiosity does increase with age among older adults (65+; Idler & Kasl, 1997). The normal development of the aging process, as well as health crises, foreground the meaning and purpose of one's life (Erikson, Erikson, & Kivnick, 1986). Poor physical health (e.g., disability), especially having life-threatening diseases (e.g., malignant cancer), is positively associated with turning to religion for help with health problems (Idler, 1995).

GENERAL HEALTH EFFECTS OF RELIGION ON OLDER ADULTS

Egbert, Mickley, and Coeling (this issue) provide a detailed review of how religion has been measured. Among older adults (65+), intrinsic religiosity—such as religious coping, or the use of religion to manage stress induced by illness and hospitalization—has been found to be negatively associated with cognitive symptoms of depression (e.g., feeling hopeless, dropping interests and activities, avoiding social gatherings; Koenig et al., 1995). This finding heightens the importance of religion for older adults, because such symptoms are difficult to treat with conventional psychopharmacology (Reynolds, 1992). Among persons 75 and older, both intrinsic and extrinsic religiosity (e.g., church attendance) are significantly associated with increased morale (Koenig, Kvale, & Ferrel, 1988). Finally, both intrinsic and extrinsic religiosity have been found to reduce the risk of mortality among older adults (55+) who are in poor health (Oxman, Freeman, & Manheimer, 1995).

SPECIFIC EFFECTS OF EXTRINSIC RELIGIOSITY
ON OLDER ADULTS

Among older adults (65+), church attendance has been positively associated with better health practices (e.g., gardening, exercising, maintaining a healthy diet, not drinking or smoking), increased social activity (e.g., leisure activities, social-network ties, holiday celebrations), and greater subjective well-being (the effect of which is pronounced among the disabled), and negatively associated with depression, somatic complaints, and interpersonal problems (Blazer & Palmore, 1976; Idler & Kasl, 1997; Koenig, Hays, et al., 1999). For persons 60 and older, religious attendance has been associated with a reduced likelihood of being hospitalized, fewer hospital admissions, and fewer days of hospitalization (Koenig & Larson, 1998). In a 6-year longitudinal study of almost 4,000 individuals, older adults (65+) who attended church frequently (vs. infrequently) were less likely to die (Koenig, Hays, et al., 1999).

A meta-analysis found that, compared to younger persons, there is a stronger relation between church attendance and subjective well-being for older (vs. younger) adults (Witter, Stock, Okun, & Haring, 1985). This is especially consequential when one considers that age is positively associated with disability (i.e., having difficulty, needing help, or not being able to do activities), and disability is negatively associated with church attendance (Idler & Kasl, 1997; Levin & Vanderpool, 1991). Compared to nondisabled older adults (65+), the positive associations between religious involvement and physical- and mental-health outcomes are more pronounced for disabled elderly (Idler & Kasl, 1997). Thus, the health-protective effects of church attendance tend to increase with age, yet advancing age tends to provide barriers to attending church.

RELIGION, THE BIOPSYCHOSOCIAL MODEL OF
MEDICINE, AND PHYSICIAN–PATIENT
COMMUNICATION

Mishler (1984) argued that patients' communication is predominantly guided by Schutz's (1962) "natural" attitude, which is similar to Habermas's (1970) "symbolic" mode of consciousness. According to Mishler, in the natural attitude, "events are located and given significance with reference to one's own biographical situation and location in the world … [E]vents take on relevance from their relationship to the acting subject's interests, purposes, and plans" (p. 122). On the other hand, as a science, medicine and medical practice have been socially constructed so as to be predominantly guided by a biomedical model (Engel, 1977), which "assumes disease to be fully accounted for by deviations from the norm of measurable biological (somatic) variables" (Engel, 1977, p. 130) and excludes social, psychological, environmental, and behavioral dimensions of illness. As such, continued Mishler, physicians' communication is predominantly guided by Schutz's "scientific" attitude, where the perspective is that of a "disinterested" observer: "[E]vents in the world are not viewed within subjective coordinates of space and time, but with reference to abstract, standard, and context-free coordinates of 'objective' space and time." (p. 122).

The concern for medicine is the following: "In approaching a physician for help, a patient brings not only a physical problem but also a social context ... A patient's experience of physical problems is inseparable from the wider social context in which these problems occur" (Waitzkin, 1991, pp. 3–4). Numerous scholars have argued that health and illness are social facts as well as biological facts; that psychological, social, environmental, and behavioral aspects (e.g., work, economic security, gender, sexuality, family, marriage and partnership, the process of aging, and community) not only have interactive effects on biological (somatic) aspects, but have their own independent effects as well (Balint, 1957; Engel, 1977). Thus, effective medicine involves a biopsychosocial model of medicine (Engel, 1977), or treating "the pathology of the whole person" (Balint, 1957, p. 103). However, due to the biomedical model, combined with the physician-guided nature of medical activities (e.g., history taking) and asymmetries of power and knowledge between physicians and patients (for a review, see Robinson, 2001), a fundamental feature of physician–patient communication—a feature that is realized through myriad practices of questioning, answering, interrupting, examining, selective note taking, and so on—is the systematic inclusion of (or focus on) biomedical topics and exclusion of (or focus away from) their psycho-social contexts; this includes the process of isolating problems that emerge from psycho-sociocontexts and transforming (or medicalizing) them into technical biomedical problems (Mishler, 1984; Waitzkin, 1991).

Religion is akin to other psychosocial factors and falls squarely into the biopsychosocial model (Sloan, Bagiella, & Powell, 1999). The *Diagnostic and Statistical Manual of Mental Disorders* recognizes religion as a relevant source of emotional support or distress. In addition to affecting health, religion can shape how patients understand and enact medical directives and advice (Barnard, Dayringer, & Cassel, 1995), as well as how patients make medical decisions, especially as they pertain to chronic and terminal illness (Wennberg, 1989).

MEDICAL EDUCATION ABOUT RELIGION AND PHYSICIAN–PATIENT COMMUNICATION

The number of U.S. medical schools offering courses dealing with religion and health has increased from 4 in 1994 to almost 30 in 1997 (Levin, Larson, &

Puchalski, 1997) to over 65 in 2002 (Koenig et al., 2000). Medical education's current stance on religion can be summarized by the following six positions. First, due to the positive effects of religion on health and differences in patients' religious beliefs, needs, and attendance practices, physicians should at least be "familiar with the basic tenets regarding the meaning and purpose of human life in the major world religions as well as with religious interpretations of sickness, suffering, and death" (Barnard et al., 1995, p. 809).

Second, as advocated in contemporary textbooks on medical examination (Bates, Bickley, & Hoekelman, 1995), at least during intake histories, physicians should conduct a religious interview (Koenig, Idler, et al., 1999; McKee & Chappel, 1992; Oxman et al., 1995; Sloan et al., 1999), which involves taking account of patients' religious values, beliefs, and practices. Physicians should not inquire into patients' religious beliefs and practices to promote nonmedical agendas (Sloan et al., 1999).

Third, physicians should not "substitute [religious] beliefs or rituals for accepted diagnostic concepts or therapeutic practice" (McKee & Chappel, 1992, p. 206). The provision of prayer as a substitute for conventional medical therapy is almost universally discouraged (Post et al., 2000).

Fourth, although there may be times when it is appropriate for physicians to inquire into patients' religious beliefs and practices (e.g., the "religious interview," discussed earlier), educators tend to agree that physicians should not take any sort of lead in providing religious guidance to patients (e.g., advice regarding religious beliefs, values, and practices, including prayer; Koenig, Idler, et al., 1999). This is so even when such guidance is adjunctive to traditional medical treatments (Sloan et al., 1999). Along these lines, physicians' offices have been considered public, secular spaces that should not contain signifiers of physicians' (or any others') religious beliefs (e.g., posters, relics, etc.; Graner, 2000). When patients ask physicians to pray with them, physicians should refer them to an identified religious leader, distinct from the patient's medical team, who can provide more competent religious care (Dagi, 1995; Post et al., 2000).

Fifth, physicians should be aware of available clergy (e.g., ministers, rabbis, pastoral counselors, hospital chaplains) and their health care-related training. Physicians should be prepared to refer patients to such clergy (Barnard et al., 1995).

Sixth, although physicians should not volunteer religious guidance or encourage patients to further participate in religious communities beyond their current levels of engagement (Koenig & Larson, 1998), physicians have been encouraged to positively reinforce and facilitate patients' extant religious behaviors (Oxman et al., 1995). This is especially true for church attendance among older adults, particularly for those who are disabled (Levin & Vanderpool, 1991).

Given the current medical stance associated with communication about religion within physician–patient interactions, little is known about the actual occurrence and content of religious talk in medical encounters. Thus, this research seeks to answer four research questions:

RQ1:   With what frequency is religion raised as a topic of discussion?
RQ2:   What aspects of religion are raised as topics of discussion?
RQ3:   What proportion of religious topics are raised by physicians and patients?
RQ4:   How do religious topics emerge in interactions with physicians and how do physicians deal with the topics?

METHOD

Participants

Participants were drawn from the Geisinger Health System, a large multispecialty group practice that provides health care for more than 2 million people in 31 counties in rural Pennsylvania. Data were collected from one county and its two hospital-based internal medicine clinics. Internal medicine physicians were targeted because as compared to family practice physicians, they tend to be less intrinsically and extrinsically religious (Koenig et al., 2000) and their patients tend to be older. Seventeen internal medicine physicians were offered $50 to participate and 12 agreed (71%). Physicians were eligible if they were an MD with a specialty in internal medicine. Patients were eligible if they were (a) an adult, (b) meeting with an internal medicine physician, (c) established with (vs. new to) the practice, and (d) visiting to deal with the routine monitoring of one or more chronic problems (e.g., hypertension, diabetes, etc.; not acute, follow-up, or physical examination visits). For each participating physician, 5 to 7 ($M = 5.8$; $SD = 2.2$) randomly selected patients were offered $20 to participate and 73 out of 100 patients agreed (73%). Two patients, a nun and a pastor, were omitted because their public occupation provided differential grounds for discussing religion-related topics (resulting in a total of 71 patients).

Procedure

This study was approved by the Human-Subjects Protection Committee of both The Pennsylvania State University and Geisinger Health System. Nurses admitted all eligible patients (beginning with the first patient of the day) and escorted them to a private room where a researcher explained the study and, if patients agreed to participate, secured their written consent. Participating patients then filled out a previsit survey, after which they were escorted to a visit room and seen by a physician. Physicians and patients interacted naturally and researchers were not present during visits. Visits were videotaped with small cameras that were positioned in ceiling corners such that their view could be obstructed by an examination curtain, which was drawn when patients dressed or underwent especially private examinations. Additionally, visits were separately audiotaped with small wireless microphones. After their visit, patients were escorted to the waiting room, filled out a postvisit questionnaire, and finally were thanked and paid $20 for their participation. All data for this article were transcribed by Jeffrey D. Robinson according to Jefferson's (Atkinson & Heritage, 1984) notation system.

RESULTS

Regarding RQ1, religion was raised as a topic of discussion in 9 out of 71 visits (13%). Regarding RQ2, topics dealt with were as follows: prayer (one case), God's will (one case), and church attendance (seven cases). Regarding RQ3, in all nine cases, religious topics were initiated by patients. RQ4 is addressed through a detailed examination and analysis of specific cases.

Prayer (One Case)

Extract 1 comes from a routine checkup for a 60-year-old, high school educated, White woman who suffers from chronic back pain and depression. The patient's 35-year-old son recently died in a car accident, but is survived by his girlfriend and their 10-month-old baby. At line 1, the patient initiates a telling about the girlfriend who, during the patient's grief over her son's death, is "thuh only one thet's bein' r:otten" (line 4).

Extract 1: [P3:88–14]

```
01    PAT:  [[My son's]] Girlfriend had a baby in december [last dec]ember.
02    DOC:                                              [I see.  ]
03          (2.2)
04    PAT:  She's thuh only one thet's bein' r:otten.
05          (0.2)
06    DOC:  .tch ↑Oh↓::. ((disappointed/sympathetic voice))
07          (1.2)
08    DOC:  Rotten to:_
09    PAT:  .hh Sh:e [asked me mond]ay fer: uh:m (1.1) death certificate
10    DOC:           [ To you:, ( )    ]
11    PAT:  >to go to thuh< socia' s'curity (.) °o:ffice.°
12          (.)
```

```
13   PAT:  .hhh >An' I-< (.) I thought (0.2) I just put my baby in thuh
14         °gro:u:nd.° (0.5) an' you're a:sking me. (0.6) already.
15         (4.0)
16   DOC:  (Mm.)
17   PAT:  She took thuh baby and left when he was two months o:ld.
18         (1.6)
19   DOC:  °>W'll that< sounds° like a very difficult_ (.) situation.
20         (0.2)
21   PAT:  It is.
22   PAT:  We'll get >th[rough it.<]
23   DOC:               [ (Mm/'n) ] (.) Befo::re.
24         (1.0)
25   PAT:  Thuh lord 'll help us.
26         (.)
27   DOC:  °Is there° anything I can do to h:elp you with it?
28         (1.2)
29   PAT:  J'st pra:yers.
30         (.)
31   DOC:  °(O)kay,°
```

At line 19, the physician produces a summative, empathetic assessment of the patient's telling as embodying a hardship: "°>W'll that< sounds° like a very difficult_ (.) situation." As part of her response, the patient says, "We'll get >through it.<" (line 22), which claims that she (and presumably her husband, and possibly even her daughter-in-law) will recover from the hardship. At line 25, the patient extends her response by providing evidence for her previous claim: "Thuh lord 'll help us." By citing the "lord" as an example of the type of help she expects, the patient displays an understanding that other more concrete, or proximate, forms of help will not be efficacious. This is understood by the physician, who immediately offers to help the patient by asking: "°Is there° anything I can do to h:elp you with it?" With the word "anything," which is a negative polarity item (Horn, 1989), the physician builds the question with a preference for a "no"-type answer, and thus a presumption of her inability to help. By stressing the word "I" (denoted by the underline), which is hearably contrastive with "Thuh lord," the physician can be heard to be offering medical, versus theological, assistance. In response, the patient explicitly produces prayer as a possible form of assistance: "J'st pra:yers." (line 29). Although the physician claims to accept the patient's answer with "°(O)kay,°" (line 31), she ultimately moves on to other matters. Neither here, nor during the rest of the visit, does the physician pray with the patient or refer her to religious counseling.

There is evidence that the patient is religious. Note that the patient's "Thuh lord 'll help us." (line 25) is not a colloquial expression, such as an idiomatic expression (e.g., "Lord help us") or a response cry (Goffman, 1976) of surprise or disappointment (e.g., "Oh my Lord"), both of which might be more readily uttered by nonreligious persons. Furthermore, the patient specifically requests "pra:yers." (line 29) as a form of help. Not only is this evidence initiated and volunteered by the patient, but "prayers" are specifically requested in the face of a medical (vs. religious) offer (line 27).

God's Will (One Case)

Extract 2 comes from a routine checkup for a 68-year-old, Italian woman who suffers from chronic knee pain. During this visit, the patient claims that she is depressed from the recent death of her closest friend, who died of cancer. A discussion ensues, and at line 1, the patient is describing her late friend's generosity.

Extract 2 [P3:]

```
01    PAT:   <She gave money> away like it was unbelievable.
02           (0.4)
03    PAT:   .h [I   ke]pt tellin' her Rosa:nna I mean: why are you doing this.
04    DOC:   [(Mm)]
05    PAT:   I me[an you should] worry about yourse:lf.
06    DOC:      [Mm hm,      ]
07    DOC:   [Mm hm.]
08    PAT:   [ .hhh   ] She=says I don' have ta worry. There's
09           plenty. she says. (.) you [know.]
10    DOC:                             [Mm h]m. Mm hm.=
11    PAT:   =There's [plent ]ly for everybody.
12    DOC:            [(Mm)]
13    DOC:   .tch Oh that's nice,
14           (.)
15    DOC:   That's a that's a very generous heart the[re.]
16    PAT:                                            [ S ]o- should- (.) if
17           th[ere is a   ] God in th[is world   ]=eh should 'e have let that
18    DOC:     [Mm hm,   ]            [ Mm hm.  ]
19    PAT:   happ[en? ]
20    DOC:       [We:]ll, you kno::w_ (0.2)
21    PAT:   [Uhhh ] ((laughter))
22    DOC:   [Maybe]: in a wa:y he was giving it to someone that he knew
23           would (.) gain pleasure by giving it [to other people.]
24    PAT:                                        [I guess:.        ] I guess:.
```

Following the physician's description of the patient's late friend as "a very generous heart" (line 15), the patient initiates an explicit question, one that pursues the physician's opinion on a matter of religion: "So- should- (.) if there is a God in this world=eh should 'e have let that happen?" (lines 16–19). The patient is not smiling or laughing while asking her question, and in this sense it is asked seriously.

The patient's question—whose generic form is something along the lines of, "If God is a benevolent, omnipotent deity, why does He allow good, innocent, and virtuous people to die premature deaths"—is a common, and theologically serious, question. Although the physician's answer at lines 20 to 23 might be characterized as harmless speculation, note that it does not address the patient's question; rather, it addresses the late friend's extreme generosity. (In the physician's answer, "he" refers to God and "it" refers to money.) Neither here, nor during the rest of the visit, does the physician refer the patient to religious counseling.

Church Attendance (Seven Cases)

The remainder of the cases involved church attendance. Five themes emerged. First, as in extracts 1 and 2, patients (vs. physicians) initiate the topic. Second, patients raise the topic not for its own sake, but as a contextualizing framework in which to relate and describe somatic problems. Third, in raising the topic, patients display that church attendance is an important, extant behavior in their lives. (A parallel theme can be found in extracts 1 and 2, where patients reveal that religion or religious issues are important.) Fourth, in each case, an argument can be made that the patients' somatic problems threaten to interfere with their attending church. Fifth, in no cases did physicians make efforts to support and facilitate patients' church attendance.

Patients raised the topic of church attendance in one of two general ways. First, it was raised as part of an answer to physicians' inquiries regarding somatic problems. For example, extract 3 comes from a routine checkup for a 66-year-old, high school educated, White, female, breast cancer survivor who suffers from depression and osteoarthritis in her knees. At line 1, the physician refers to Viox, a prescription medication being used to treat the patient's arthritis.

Extract 3 [P3:95-15]

```
01   DOC:   (H)as 'at been helping at a:ll? ((referring to Viox))
02    PAT:   Oh a little. not_ (0.7) not all <that much.>
03   DOC:   Are you stiff when you first go da get up outta thuh cha:ir,
04           an' things,
05   DOC:   Ye:ah,
06           (0.5)
07   DOC:   Ooh::. ((sympathetic voice))
08           (0.4)
09    PAT:   I have ta (0.2) I have ta get up_ (.) with both a my ha:nds o:n
10           thuh chair. Even in [church.]
```

```
11  DOC:                        [Mm:.  ]
12          (0.2)
13  PAT:  When I'm in church even ta stand up at church I °'ave° ta pu:ll.
14          (.)
15  PAT:  Pull my self up.
16          (.)
17  PAT:  I [can't_ (.)] get up_
18  DOC:    [Mm/Hm ]
19          (.)
20  DOC:  Okay,
21          (.)
22  PAT:  C[an't      ca]rry anything up thuh stairs any more,
23  DOC:    [(Do y' w-)]
24  DOC:  Have ya tried takin' ↑two of thuh vi:↓ox.
25  PAT:  No.
```

At line 2, the patient communicates that her current dosage of Viox is not providing sufficient relief. At lines 3 to 4, perhaps to more fully understand the patient's answer and condition, the physician pursues his initial question by asking
the patient to confirm or disconfirm a generic scenario: "Are you stiff when you
first go da get up outta thuh cha:ir, an' things." Simultaneous with the word
"cha:ir," the patient begins a confirmatory head nod; from this point through line 6,
the patient produces two nods in one continuous motion. After the patient's initial
head nod, the physician pursues confirmation with "Ye:ah," to which he receives
another head nod. At line 7, the physician sympathetically and negatively assesses
the patient's condition with "Ooh::." The physician's assessment possibly closes
the question–answer sequence at lines 1 to 6 (Schegloff, 1995). During the silence
at line 8, the physician returns his gaze to the patient's medical records. At line 9,
the patient initiates a turn of talk wherein she continues to answer the physician's
question at lines 3 to 4—here, she upgrades the severity of her condition by mov-
ing from a simple confirmation of the physician's medical description "stiff" to the
provision of a more severe description: "I have ta get up_ (.) with both a my ha:nds
o:n thuh chair" (lines 9–10).The patient immediately continues to extend her explanation of the severity of her condition by adding the following: "Even in
church" (line 10). At lines 10 to 17, the patient moves beyond the physician's generic scenario and contextualizes her arthritic condition—specifically, her problem with standing from a sitting position—within the activity of church attendance. After passing on at least four interactional places where it would have been
relevant to acknowledge, or otherwise respond to, the patient's church scenario
(i.e., lines 12, 14, 16, and 19), the physician finally does so with "Okay," (line 20).
The physician maintains his previous biomedical agenda by proceeding to ask an-

other question: "Have ya tried takin' ↑two of thuh vi:↓ox" (line 24). Neither here, nor during the rest of the visit, does the physician deal with church attendance.

For a second example, see extract 4, which comes from a routine checkup for an 83-year-old, 10th-grade-educated, White man who suffers from irritable bowel syndrome, degenerative back disease, coronary artery disease, and anxiety.

Extract 4 [P3:011-03]

```
01   DOC:   Okay bo:wels >that was thee other< thing we follow is that
02          irritable bowel (h)as that been doin'_ (0.2) okay er
03   PAT:   d-=Oh::: yes sir. ( ) (.) °°(is better)°°
04   PAT:   B't sunday is ba:d. I(h) d(h)on't k(h)now why sunday, I
05          [said I'm ] going ta church- sunday school if it (k)- if I gotta
06   DOC:   [Oh yeah,]
07   PAT:   go on my hands an' knees. I: went. .hh an' (nen) then: I: uh:
08          felt a little better, an' [.hh]
09   DOC:                        [N ]k[ay.   ]
10   PAT:                             [°b't°] it- it- (0.2) gr-=I: I
11          'ave good da:ys an' bad days. that's all I can say.
12   DOC:   A'right;
```

In response to the physician's question regarding the irritable bowel, "(h)as that been doin'_ (0.2) okay" (line 2), the patient responds affirmatively, "yes sir." (line 3). Following some unintelligible talk (line 3, denoted by the parentheses), the patient continues his turn by hedging his previously unproblematic assessment with a piece of contrasting evidence: "B't sunday is ba:d." (line 4). The patient continues to explicate his assessment "ba:d" by reporting his response to the pain, a response that is grounded in a concrete event (i.e., church attendance): "I said I'm going ta church- sunday school if it (k)- if I gotta go on my hands an' knees" (lines 4–7). The patient's response simultaneously displays his perception of the importance of church and of the threat his medical condition poses to such attendance.

A third example, seen in extract 5, comes from a routine checkup for a 46-year-old, high school educated, White, female secretary who suffers from diabetes and, recently, knee pain.

Extract 5 [P3:060-10]

```
01   DOC:   You're having knee problems since (.) Ju:ne.
02   PAT:   Yes.
                    .
             . ((physician takes history of knee; six questions omitted))
                    .
03   DOC:   .hhh It does not restrict your <physical_> (.) capabilities.
04          you're still able to do: >whatever you< normally feel like.
```

```
05   PAT:  The only thing I can't do I can't get down=on=my knee to
06          scrub my floor anymore.
07   DOC:  Okay,
08   PAT:  An' I can't kneel in church anymore.
09          (.)
10   DOC:  Okay;
11          (1.0)
12   DOC:  Ah=h have you noticed any swelling in thuh joint,
```

As part of a series of questions about the patient's "knee problems" (line 1), the physician addresses its effects on her "<physical_> (.) capabilities" (line 3), and requests confirmation that: "you're still able to do: >whatever you< normally feel like" (line 4). This question specifically addresses the relation between the medical problem and what Engel (1977) termed "problems of living," and the patient responds by relating that her knee problems interfere with her ability to do housework (lines 5–6). The physician acknowledges the patient's answer with "Okay" (line 7). Insofar as the patient communicated that this was "The only thing" (line 5), the physician's "Okay" (line 7) possibly closes the question–answer sequence and projects a shift to a new question or action (Beach, 1995). However, the patient continues to produce a second restriction: "An' I can't kneel in church anymore" (line 8). This is also acknowledged by the physician and, after a long silence (line 11), the physician reasserts his biomedical agenda (begun at line 1) by asking a new question about the patient's knee (line 12).

Patients do not have to capitalize on physicians' questions to raise the topic of church attendance. In two cases, patients simply initiate a complaint that implicates church attendance. For example, see extract 6, which comes from a routine checkup for a 76-year-old, high school educated, retired, White man who suffers from back pain, high blood pressure, diabetes, and coronary heart disease.

Extract 6 [P3:169-26]

```
01   DOC:  How's your brea:thing.
02          (0.4)
03   PAT:  Goo:d. (0.2) goo:d.
04   DOC:  (N)ka(:y)
05          (0.2)
06   PAT:  Good.
07          (.)
08   PAT:  No:w uh:_ (.) .hhhhhhhhhh ((1.0)) hh=uh::=hhhh {(w- w-) / (0.4)}
09          How should I=s tell ya this. .hh When I go da church_ (0.2) say
10          I'm in church.
11   DOC:  Mm hm::,
12   PAT:  Okay, (.) .h 'f I'm settin' there. (1.2) an' all of a sudden_ (.)
```

```
13           we have ta get up.
14           (.)
15  DOC:  Mm hm[:,      ]
16  PAT:        [You kn]o:w
17           (0.4)
18  DOC:  You feel a little light headed [when you get [up.]
19  PAT:                                 [ I::         [get] dizzy
20           a[s hel  ]l.
21  DOC:     [(Mm:)]
22           (.)
23           ???: .hhh
24  DOC:  You [have to get up] s[l_o_:_:]w.
25  PAT:      [So::          ]  [what (I)]
26  PAT:  W- Yeah. well what I do I (.) lean on thuh (0.2) on thuh pew
27           next_ (0.4) in fron' a me.
28           (0.7)
29  PAT:  A:n'_ (0.2) <until> it_ (.) goes awa:y. which is a couple a .hh
30           'bout half a minute or so maybe,
31           (3.0)
32  PAT:  But duh=hh (1.8) I guess that's normal, I don't know.
33           (0.4)
34  DOC:  We::ll (.) unfortunately that's (.) probably:=uh:m (.) part of
35           your diabetes.
```

At line 1, the physician asks for an assessment of one of the patient's chronic problems, "How's your brea:thing" (line 1), to which the patient responds positively: "Goo:d. (0.2) goo:d." (line 3). The physician's subsequent "(N)ka(:y)" (line 4) acknowledges the patient's answer, possibly closes the question–answer sequence, and projects a shift to new matters (Beach, 1995). However, the patient continues to reiterate his positive assessment, "Good" (line 6) and, after a brief silence (line 7), initiates a new topic dealing with a different problem: lightheadedness when standing up (which is likely caused by his diabetes, although the patient does not realize this). The patient initially, and explicitly, struggles with how to describe his problem: "How should I=s tell ya this" (line 9). The patient's solution is to contextualize his problem in the activity of church attendance: "When I go da church_ (0.2) say I'm in church." (lines 9–10). In overlap with the physician's remedy, "You have to get up slo::w." (line 24), the patient begins to describe his solution, "So:: what (I) … " (line 25), which he completes at line 30. During the long silence at line 31, the physician reads the patient's medical records. If the patient orients to his lightheadedness as a relatively new problem, then his presentation of the problem may have made relevant some sort of diagnosis by the physician (Robinson, 2003), which is absent during the silence at line 31.

This argument is supported by the fact that the patient continues to pursue a diagnosis, "But duh=hh (1.8) I guess that's normal, I don't know." (line 32; Robinson, 2001), and the physician responds by providing one: "that's (.) probably:=uh:m () part of your diabetes" (lines 33–34).

For a second example, see extract 7, which comes from a routine checkup for an 87-year-old, seventh-grade-educated, retired, White woman who suffers from incontinence and chronic back pain. The patient is homebound by her medical conditions and assisted by a part-time nurse. During the following extract, the physician is physically examining the patient, who is sitting on the exam table. (The patient's daughter, "DAU," is also in the room.)

Extract 7 [P3:056-10]

```
01   DOC:   (Gunna) look in your e:ars.
02          (6.0)
03   PAT:   They itch so.
04          (4.0)
05   DOC:   Well you got some wax buildup on this si:de,
06          (4.0)
07   PAT:   (Then) my ey:es itch too:.
08          (15.0)
09   PAT:   (Then) my <'fridgerator> wen' o:ut.
10   DAU:   Huh heh (.) heh heh,
11   PAT:   Huh
12          (.)
13   PAT:   (That's it.)
14          (0.2)
15   DOC:   Not=a been=a good week for you.
16   PAT:   u=N:o en=eh (.) good two da::ys. °(huh)°
17          (7.0)
18   PAT:   My priest ca:lled ta bring communion.
19          (.)
20   PAT:   I said £oh: no:.£
21          (1.4)
22   PAT:   Tomarrah, (1.1) (s)o he's commin' 'ommorro[w.]
23   DOC:                                            [ U]h huh,
24          (0.2)
25   DOC:   °Ukay°,
26   DOC:   Let me listen to your heart here,
```

At lines 3 and 7, the patient produces two complaints regarding physical symptoms (i.e. her ears and eyes itch). After 15 sec of silent examination (line 8), the patient produces another complaint, this time shifting from the realm of physical symptoms to that of daily living: "(Then) my <'fridgerator> wen' o:ut." (line 9). Although the physician does not cease his examination, he does sympathize with the patient—at line 15, he formulates an upshot of at least the patient's complaint about her refrigerator (and perhaps about the patient's multiple complaints) by characterizing her as having had a bad week, to which the patient agrees. Line 17 constitutes another 7 sec of silent examination. Out of this silence, the patient initiates a second complaint in the realm of daily living: "My priest ca:lled ta bring communion" (line 18). This homebound patient's priest had called to schedule a time for communion that conflicted with her present appointment with the physician. There is evidence that the patient orients to this as a complaint in her report of how she responded to the potential conflict: "I said £oh: no:.£" (line 20). The patient's "oh:" displays that she had not anticipated the conflict (Heritage, 1984), and the rejection component "no:" displays her understanding of the conflict as being undesirable. This is further supported by the fact that the patient reports rescheduling the visit for "Tomarrah" (line 22). This is acknowledged by the physician with "Uh huh" (line 23), who then proceeds to project a shift to a new examination, "°Ukay°," (Beach, 1995), which he does at line 26.

DISCUSSION

Church attendance is a unique and prevalent aspect of social support, especially for older adults, and is associated with myriad positive health outcomes. Despite this, there are several reasons why it can be ethically and practically inappropriate for physicians to initiate and provide religious "guidance" to patients, including praying with patients and advising patients to practice previously nonpracticed religious behaviors (e.g., church attendance). The primary reason is that, due to physicians' role or relationship with patients—that is, the asymmetrical power, status, and emotional- and physical-needs relationship (Parsons, 1975)—physicians' religious guidance can be unduly influential (McKee & Chappel, 1992; Oxman et al., 1995). This is complicated by the religious gap between physicians and patients, with physicians being less intrinsically and extrinsically religious than the general population (Maugans & Wadland, 1991). Another reason is that many physicians are not professionally competent in the provision of religious care and advice. Finally, despite their enormous benefits, intrinsic and extrinsic religiosity have also been associated with negative health outcomes (Ellison & Levin, 1998).

There are at least two types of evidence that researchers, educators, and physicians have used to justify initiating and discussing religious issues. First, according to national statistics, a significant majority of the U.S. population reports a belief in God (96%), and a large minority (42%) report that they attend regular religious services. Second, a number of studies have revealed that a majority (80%–93%) of patients report that primary-care physicians should "consider" patients' religious needs (King & Bushwick, 1994; King, Sobal, Haggerty, Dent, & Patton, 1992). Ethically, however, neither reason warrants physicians initiating and discussing religious issues. National rates of belief in God and church attendance vary dramatically by geographic location. Furthermore, research has found that a majority of patients (79%) disagree that physicians have the "responsibility" to make religious inquiries, and that only a minority of patients (albeit a large minority; 40%–48%) report that they would like their physicians to address or discuss religious issues (Maugans & Wadland, 1991), pray with them (King & Bushwick, 1994), or discuss personal religious beliefs more (King & Bushwick, 1994). Overall, there are numerous ethical hazards associated with initiating and providing religious guidance that dissuade physicians from making inquiries.

In light of these ethical hazards, medical education encourages physicians to reinforce or facilitate patients' "extant" religious behaviors, particularly church attendance. One barrier to enacting this pedagogy is that physicians rarely know about patients' "extant" religious behaviors. As such, physicians are encouraged to ask about such behaviors in a "religious interview." However, this rarely happens (Maugans & Wadland, 1991), and when it does, it typically occurs during an intake interview and in a manner that is divorced from particular medical problems or concerns (e.g., "Do you attend church?" "How frequently?"). Without results from a religious interview, the biomedical model biases physicians (psychologically and interactionally) away from addressing, and perhaps even considering, psychosocial aspects of patients' somatic concerns, including religion. Indeed, a majority of physicians (51%), report that patients rarely or never mention religion (Koenig, Bearon, & Dayringer, 1989), and it has been speculated that "[u]nless a physician overtly or tacitly invites comments about spiritual and religious interests, patients may seldom mention them" (Koenig, Moberg, & Kvale, 1988, p. 363). Importantly, but perhaps not surprisingly, given more recent research on ways in which patients solicit information and initiate topics (Robinson, 2001), the aforementioned research, reports, and speculations are contraindicated by the present findings.

In this data, the topic of religion was raised in 13% of the visits, and in every single one of these cases, the topic of religion was volunteered by patients. Thirteen percent of visits may seem low compared to prior findings regarding the frequency of discussing other so-called lifestyle topics, such as smoking (43%–81%), drinking (19%–69%), exercise (40%–56%), and nutrition (26%–56%; Bertakis & Callahan, 1992; Johanson, Larsson, Saljo, & Svardsudd, 1995). However, these topics are relatively closely tied to biomedical aspects of health, whereas topics with more distant ties such as housing arrangements (7%), stress (5%), and sexual habits (7%) are discussed much less frequently (Johanson et al., 1995). Thus, in comparison to these latter lifestyle topics, religion (13%) appears to be a relatively common topic in physician–patient communication.

In cases 1 to 5 of this study, patients raised the topic or religion as part of a response to a physician-initiated utterance that made a response relevant. In cases 6 to 7, patients voluntarily initiated utterances that contained topics related to church attendance. In each case, however, patients used an aspect of religion to ground, or contextualize, relatively abstract problems in concrete, lived aspects of their social lives. In cases 1 and 3 to 5, patients literally worked interactively to transition from a purely biomedical frame to one with psychosocial implications. That is, physicians' questions were addressed to patients' somatic or medical–psychological problems (e.g., knee pain or depression), and patients' initial answers responded to, and within, the biomedical frames of the questions. However, patients continued to expand their initial answers, beyond places where physicians were interactionally within their rights to take the floor, to ground their initial answers in a religious aspect of their social lives. All of these observations support a basic tenet of the biopsychosocial model of medicine, which is that patients' physical problems are inseparable from their social contexts. These observations also highlight Balint's early observation: "[I]f the doctor asks questions in the manner of medical history-taking, he will always get answers—but hardly anything more. Before he can arrive at what we called 'deeper' diagnosis, he has to learn to listen" (Balint, 1957, p. 121, emphasis deleted). Du Pre (2002) argued that patients often gauge how sick they are by the affect of their illness on their social activities. When patients contextualize their problems in aspects of their religious lives—and especially when patients explicitly orient to the personal importance of religious activities, such as church attendance—patients' revelations solve the predicament of pedagogy mentioned earlier. That is, patients themselves reveal their "extant" religious behaviors. Furthermore, the "validity" of such revelations are high insofar as they are not abstract answers to decontextualized religious-interview questions, but rather utterances that are concretely and intimately linked to lived moments in patients' lives.

CONCLUSIONS

In sum, there are numerous pressures working against physician-initiated inquiries into patients' religious behaviors, and without such information, physicians are practically unable, and ethically ill advised, to facilitate or reinforce such behaviors. This ethical and practical predicament of pedagogy is resolved, at least in part, if patients themselves reveal their extant religious behaviors or beliefs, and thus indirectly (or directly) reveal their commitment to such behaviors or beliefs. In other words, if patients initiate a topic that reveals their commitment or desire to attend church, as 13% of participants did in this study, they metaphorically open the ethical and topical door for physicians to facilitate and reinforce such attendance. Future research should strive to further inform our understanding of the biopsychosocial model of medicine and should provide solutions to the practical and ethical bias posed by medical education in terms of physicians addressing religion.

REFERENCES

Atkinson, J. M., & Heritage, J. (Eds.). (1984). *Structures of social action: Studies in conversation analysis.* Cambridge, England: Cambridge University Press.

Balint, M. (1957). *The doctor, his patient, and the illness.* New York: International Universities Press.

Baltes, P. B., & Baltes, M. M. (1990). *Successful aging: Perspectives from the behavioral sciences.* New York: Cambridge University Press.

Barnard, D., Dayringer, R., & Cassel, C. K. (1995). Toward a person-centered medicine: Religious studies in the medical curriculum. *Academic Medicine, 70,* 806–812.

Barrera, M. (1986). Distinctions between social support concepts, measures, and models. *American Journal of Community Psychology, 14,* 413–445.

Bates, B., Bickley, L. S., & Hoekelman, R. A. (1995). *Physical examination and history taking* (6th ed.). Philadelphia: Lippincott.

Beach, W. A. (1995). Preserving and constraining options: "Okays" and 'official' priorities in medical interviews. In B. Morris & R. Chenail (Eds.), *Talk of the clinic* (pp. 259–289). Hillsdale, NJ: Lawrence Erlbaum Associates, Inc.

Beisecker, A. E., & Thompson, T. L. (1995). The elderly patient–physician interaction. In J. F. Nussbaum & J. Coupland (Eds.), *Handbook of communication and aging research* (pp. 397–416). Hillsdale, NJ: Lawrence Erlbaum Associates, Inc.

Bertakis, K. D., & Callahan, E. J. (1992). A comparison of initial and established patient encounters using the Davis observation code. *Family Medicine, 24,* 307–311.

Blazer, D., & Palmore, E. (1976). Religion and aging in a longitudinal panel. *The Gerontologist, 16,* 82–85.

Dagi, T. F. (1995). Prayer, piety, and professional propriety: Limits on religious expression in hospitals. *Journal of Clinical Ethics, 6,* 274–279.

Du Pre, A. (2002). Accomplishing the impossible: Talking about body and soul and mind during a medical visit. *Health Communication, 14,* 1–21.

Durkheim, E. (1951). *Suicide: A study in sociology.* New York: Free Press.

Ellison, C. G., & Levin, J. S. (1998). The religion–health connection: Evidence, theory, and future directions. *Health Education and Behavior, 25,* 700–720.

Engel, G. L. (1977). The need for a new medical model: A challenge for biomedicine. *Science, 196,* 129–196.

Erikson, E. H., Erikson, J. M., & Kivnick, H. Q. (1986). *Vital involvement in old age.* New York: Norton.

Goffman, E. (1976). Replies and responses. *Language in Society, 5,* 257–313.

Graner, J. (2000). Letters: Physicians and patient spirituality. *Annals of Internal Medicine, 133,* 748.

Habermas, J. (1970). Toward a theory of communicative competence. In H. P. Dreitzel (Ed.), *Recent sociology no. 2* (pp. 114–148). New York: Macmillian.

Heritage, J. (1984). A change-of-state token and aspects of its sequential placement. In J. M. Atkinson & J. Heritage (Eds.), *Structures of social action* (pp. 299–345). Cambridge, England: Cambridge University Press.

Horn, L. (1989). *A natural history of negation.* Chicago: University of Chicago Press.

House, J. S., Landis, K. R., & Umberson, D. (1988). Social relationships and health. *Science, 241,* 540–545.

Idler, E. L. (1995). Religion, health, and nonphysical senses of self. *Social Forces, 74,* 683–704.

Idler, E. L., & Kasl, S. V. (1997). Religion among disabled and nondisabled persons I: Cross-sectional patterns in health practices, social activities, and well-being. *Journal of Gerontology, 52B*, S294–S305.

James, W. (1978). *The varieties of religious experience.* New York: Image Books.

Johanson, M., Larsson, U. S., Saljo, R., & Svardsudd, K. (1995). Lifestyle in primary health care discourse. *Social Science and Medicine, 40*, 339–348.

King, D. E., & Bushwick, B. (1994). Beliefs and attitudes of hospital inpatients about faith healing and prayer. *Journal of Family Practice, 39*, 349–352.

King, D. E., Sobal, J., Haggerty, J., Dent, M., & Patton, D. (1992). Experiences and attitudes about faith healing among family physicians. *Journal of Family Practice, 35*, 158–162.

Koenig, H. G., Bearon, L. B., & Dayringer, R. (1989). Physician perspectives on the role of religion in the physician–older patient relationship. *Journal of Family Practice, 28*, 441–448.

Koenig, H. G., Cohen, H. J., Blazer, D. G., Kudler, H. S., Krishnan, K. R. R., & Sibert, T. E. (1995). Religious coping and cognitive symptoms of depression in elderly medical patients. *Psychosomatics, 36*, 369–375.

Koenig, H. G., Hays, J. C., Larson, D. B., George, L. K., Cohen, H. J., McCullough, M. E., et al. (1999). Does religious attendance prolong survival? A six-year follow-up study of 3,968 older adults. *Journal of Gerontology, 54A*, M370–M376.

Koenig, H. G., Idler, E. L., Stanislav, K., Hays, J. C., George, L. K., Musick, M., et al. (1999). Religion, spirituality, and medicine: A rebuttal to skeptics. *International Journal of Psychiatry in Medicine, 29*, 123–131.

Koenig, H. G., Kvale, J. N., & Ferrel, C. (1988). Religion and well-being in later life. *The Gerontologist, 28*, 18–28.

Koenig, H. G., & Larson, D. B. (1998). Use of hospital services, religious attendance, and religious affiliation. *Southern Medical Journal, 91*, 925–932.

Koenig, H. G., McCullough, M. E., & Larson, D. B. (2000). *Religion and health: A century of research reviewed.* New York: Oxford University Press.

Koenig, H. G., Moberg, D. O., & Kvale, J. N. (1988). Religious activities and attitudes of older adults in a geriatric assessment clinic. *Journal of the American Geriatric Society, 36*, 362–374.

Krause, N. (2001). Social support. In R. H. Binstock & L. K. George (Eds.), *Handbook of aging and the social sciences* (5th ed., pp. 272–294). San Diego, CA: Academic.

Krause, N., Morgan, D., Chatters, L., & Meltzer, T. (2000). Using focus groups to explore the nature of prayer in later life. *Journal of Aging Studies, 14*, 191–212.

Levin, J. S. (1996). How religion influences morbidity and health: Reflections on natural history, salutogenesis and host resistance. *Social Science and Medicine, 43*, 849–864.

Levin, J. S. (2001). *God, faith, and health: Exploring the spirituality–healing connection.* New York: Wiley.

Levin, J. S., Larson, D. B., & Puchalski, C. M. (1997). Religion and spirituality in medicine: Research and education. *Journal of the American Medical Association, 278*, 792–793.

Levin, J. S., & Vanderpool, H. Y. (1991). Religious factors in physical health and the prevention of illness. Binghamton, NY: Haworth.

Maugans, T. A., & Wadland, W. C. (1991). Religion and family medicine: A survey of physicians and patients. *Journal of Family Practice, 32*, 210–213.

McFadden, S. H. (1995). Religion and well-being in aging persons in an aging society. *Journal of Social Issues, 51*(2), 161–175.

McKee, D. D., & Chappel, J. N. (1992). Spirituality and medical practice. *Journal of Family Practice, 35*, 201–208.

Mills, P. J. (2002). Spirituality, religiousness, and health: From research to clinical practice. *Annals of Behavioral Medicine, 1*, 1–2.

Mishler, E. (1984). *The discourse of medicine: Dialectics of medical interviews.* Norwood, NJ: Ablex.

Norris, F. H., & Kaniasty, K. (1996). Received and perceived social support in times of stress: A test of the social support deterioration deterrence model. *Journal of Personality and Social Psychology, 71,* 498–511.

Nussbaum, J. F., Pecchioni, L. L., Baringer, D. K., & Kundrat, A. L. (2002). Lifespan communication. In W. B. Gudykunst (Ed.), *Communication Yearbook 26* (pp. 366–389). Mahwah, NJ: Lawrence Erlbaum Associates, Inc.

Nussbaum, J. F., Pecchioni, L. L., Robinson, J. D., & Thompson, T. L. (2000). *Communication and aging* (2nd ed.). Mahwah, NJ: Lawrence Erlbaum Associates, Inc.

Oxman, T. E., Freeman, D. H., & Manheimer, E. D. (1995). Lack of social participation or religious strength and comfort as risk factors for death after cardiac surgery in the elderly. *Psychosomatic Medicine, 57,* 5–15.

Parsons, T. (1975). The sick role and the role of the physician reconsidered. *Milbank Memorial Fund Quarterly, 53,* 257–278.

Post, S. G., Puchalski, C. M., & Larson, D. B. (2000). Physicians and patient spirituality: Professional boundaries, competency, and ethics. *Annual Journal of Internal Medicine, 132*(7), 578–583.

Reynolds, C. F. (1992). Treatment of depression in special populations. *Journal of Clinical Psychiatry, 53,* 45–53.

Robinson, J. (2001). Asymmetry in action: Sequential resources in the negotiation of a prescription request. *Text, 21,* 19–54.

Robinson, J. (2003). An interactional structure of medical activities during acute visits and its implications for patients' participation. *Health Communication, 15,* 27–59.

Roter, D. (2000). The enduring and evolving nature of the patient–physician relationship. *Patient Education and Counseling, 39,* 5.

Schegloff, E. A. (1995). *Sequence organization.* Unpublished manuscript.

Schutz, A. (1962). *Collected papers, volume 1: The problem of social reality.* The Hague, The Netherlands: Martinus Nijhoff.

Sloan, R. P., Bagiella, E., & Powell, T. (1999). Religion, spirituality, and medicine. *The Lancet, 353,* 664–667.

Vanderpool, H. Y., & Levin, J. S. (1990). Religion and medicine: How are they related? *Journal of Religion Health, 29,* 9–17.

Waitzkin, H. (1991). *The politics of medical encounters.* New Haven, CT: Yale University Press.

Wennberg, R. N. (1989). *Terminal choices: Euthanasia, suicide, and the right to die.* Grand Rapids, Michigan: Eerdmans.

Witter, R. A., Stock, W. A., Okun, M. A., & Haring, M. J. (1985). Religion and subjective well-being in adulthood: A quantitative synthesis. *Review of Religious Research, 26,* 332–341.

Final Conversations: Survivors' Memorable Messages Concerning Religious Faith and Spirituality

Maureen P. Keeley

Department of Communication Studies
Texas State University–San Marcos

This article reports on the findings from a project exploring final conversations (FCs). The FC project examines communication with the terminally ill from the often-overlooked survivor's perspective ($N = 30$). The researcher focuses purposely on one major theme discovered in the FC interviews, that of messages shared regarding religious faith or spirituality. Messages pertaining to religious faith or spirituality were identified in 26 of the 30 FC interviews. The results revealed that validation-comfort and validation-community were the dominant themes in FC. Further, when framed as memorable messages, these FC excerpts revealed three "rules of conduct" relating to the following: (a) how to cope with life's challenges after a loved one is gone, (b) how to be involved in the death and dying process, and (c) how to enact or live your religion or spirituality. Implications for health communication theory and research, as well as comforting literature, are discussed.

Kubler-Ross's (1969) groundbreaking work on death and dying established the need for communication between the terminally ill person and family. The majority of research on end-of-life communication, however, focuses on the importance of communication from the dying person's perspective (Aiken, 2001; Callanan & Kelley, 1992). Communication at the end-of-life is also important for the surviving family members and close friends, impacting their health and well-being (Nadeau, 1998). Family members seek opportunities for final communication with the dying loved one (Gold, 1984), expressing concerns similar to those expressed by the dying person (Fieweger & Smilowitz, 1984). Especially important to people facing death, be it their own or a loved one's, is the search for meaning, the examination of

---

Requests for reprints should be sent to Maureen P. Keeley, Department of Communication Studies, Texas State University–San Marcos, San Marcos, TX 78666. E-mail: mk09@txstate.edu

religious belief systems, an exploration of spirituality, and a consideration of personal philosophies (Marrone, 1999). People begin this process through communication during final conversations (FC) with dying loved ones, following confirmation of a terminal illness. Communication at the end of life from the survivor's perspective is an overlooked health communication issue. A broad arena with significant unanswered questions, this article begins the process of examining FC by exploring the emergence of discourse relating to religious faith and spirituality.

TALK ABOUT RELIGIOUS FAITH AND SPIRITUALITY IN THE FACE OF DEATH AND GRIEF

There is a great deal to learn about issues revolving around communication about religious faith and spirituality in the face of a loved one's death, including how the health and quality of life of survivors may be impacted (Marrone, 1999). Leis, Kristjanson, Koop, and Laizner (1997) concurred, suggesting that research explore the effects of spirituality on families' experiences with terminal illness. In the literature on death and bereavement, the terms *religion* and *spirituality* are often used interchangeably (Pargament, 1999), but may be distinguished in the following ways:

> Religiousness has specific behavioral, social, doctrinal, and denominational characteristics because it involves a system of worship and doctrine that is shared within a group. Spirituality is concerned with transcendent, addressing ultimate questions about life's meaning, with the assumption that there is more to life than what we see or fully understand. (Underwood & Teresi, 2002, p. 23)

Religious or spiritual beliefs often provide family members a consoling explanation for events that cannot be explained by reference to science and logic alone (Davis & Nolen–Hoeksema, 2001; Dull & Skokan, 1995). People that have religious or spiritual beliefs are likely to be less anxious about death (McKenzie, 1980). In fact, when people face death, they often begin a religious or spiritual quest (Gentile & Fello, 1990; Heinz, 1999). The dying person's loved ones are also searching for meaning, and religious faith or spirituality is a critical component to their ability to ascribe meaning to loss (Davis & Nolen–Hoeksema, 2001). How these spiritual searches emerge in conversations between those facing death and their loved ones has rarely been examined. Palliative care nurses have described resistance, denial, unrealistic optimism, and anger as blocks to open communication with the dying (McGrath, Yates, Clinton, & Hart, 1999), which may also inhibit discussion about death between the dying and their loved ones.

Three principal tasks associated with dying have been identified, with extrapolation of these tasks to the experiences of friends and family demonstrating great relevance (Doka, 1993). One task is to find the meaning or significance of life, with answers possibly found in religious or spiritual beliefs and an inability to find answers producing deep feelings of spiritual anguish. A second task is to evolve an appropriate framework to accept death in a way that is consistent with individual values and lifestyles, with religious faith and spirituality guiding the formation of thoughts to accommodate death as part of life. Third, people need to transcend death, which may be accomplished through new spiritual insights, a renewed promise of eternal life gained from religious doctrine, or assurances that their deeds will continue after they die.

Both those with religious faith and spirituality as guiding frameworks and those without such frames search for personal meaning when faced with a love one's death, looking for the benefits gained from the experience. The three most common benefits reported include a strengthening of relationships or increased sense of connectedness with others, a growth in character, and a gain in perspective (Nolen-Hoeksema & Larson, 1999). Communication research suggests the validity of asserting that FC will be the site of "strengthening of relationships" during the period of the terminal illness. Discussing intimate issues such as "confronting the past, speaking the unspeakable, acknowledging the difficult, and talking about death can lead to the development of an intimate relationship" (Nussbaum, Pecchioni, Robinson, & Thompson, 2000, p. 44). Second, "a growth in character" is often the result of being affected by the death process. Approximately three decades have passed since Marshall (1975) found that being around death, experiencing loss, and observing how to address these events help people prepare for their own eventual death. Third, communication is a necessary component for the attainment of a "gain in perspective." FitzSimmons (1994) suggested that talking about the death experience helps to clarify feelings for all participants while putting death into perspective. An additional benefit of talking about death is that the talks help all participants deal with their emotions (FitzSimmons, 1994; P. R. Silverman, Weiner, & El Ad, 1995). These meanings are "often intensely personal and perhaps to some extent nonverbal ... and are no doubt ... tested and revised, at least subtly, in interactions with others" (Davis & Nolen-Hoeksema, 2001, p. 737). How religious faith and spirituality emerge in these conversations, especially prior to the passing of a loved one, is not known. Prior theorizing and research within communication suggest that their role will be a significant one. Thus, the first research question that this article addresses follows:

RQ1: What major themes pertaining to spirituality or religiosity emerge from FCs?

MEMORABLE MESSAGES FRAMEWORK

Interpersonal messages that are remembered for a long time and have a significant effect on a person's life are identified as "memorable messages" (Knapp, Stohl, & Reardon, 1981). Memorable messages often have a profound impact on a person's life because they are "internalized" and "taken to heart" (Knapp et al., 1981, p. 39). According to Knapp et al., a number of factors contribute to whether an interpersonal message becomes a memorable one. First, the event where the interaction occurred is usually a single, significant episode in the person's life or there is something unique about the event. Memorable messages are most often received from a person who was held in great esteem. The messages are usually brief, have a personal focus, and the conversation occurs at a time when the person is seeking something (therefore, perceptual and emotional receptivity is high). Last, they have a relatively simple rule structure. Given the aforementioned criteria, FC about religious faith and spirituality are likely to be memorable messages. Having a FC with a close loved one (be it a parent, spouse, sibling, grandparent, close friend, etc.) is easily construed as a significant and distinctive event in a person's life. In fact, usually, the dying person has gatekeepers around to insure that only close family and friends are given access to the person that is dying, thereby acknowledging the importance of the interaction between the participants of the FC. Second, the dying person is often held in great esteem because of the type of relationship (e.g., parent–child, grandparent–grandchild, etc.), the nature of the relationship (e.g., a close and intimate relationship), or the realization that the FC may be the last message that is received from the dying person. Third, because the dying person often does not feel well, is tired, or may be incapable of sustaining a long conversation, many messages found in FC are brief (Callanan & Kelley, 1992). Fourth, the messages exchanged in FC that are memorable often have a very personal focus because the presence of a significant life challenge such as a terminal illness usually forces people to reassess what is important, and what is often discovered is that what matters most is the relationships in peoples' lives (Lynn, Harrold, & the Center to Improve Care for the Dying, 1999). Fifth, the person who must go on living after the death of a loved one is very receptive to messages as a way to make sense of their loss and their experience. People are often looking to learn something new about themselves or about the value of relationships as a way to come to terms with the death and loss of their loved one (Davis & Nolen-Hoeksema, 2001). Sixth, the communicative structure of FC is likely to be simple, due in large part to physical or mental constraints experienced by the dying person (Callanan & Kelley, 1992). Thus, a memorable message perspective provides a valuable framework from which to analyze religious discourse from FC.

According to Knapp et al. (1981), memorable messages usually prescribe "rules of conduct" or specify personal, action-oriented advice enabling the person to solve personal problems. "The memorable message may be one which 'makes everything clear' in retrospect or it may be a message which has over the years, represented a superordinate injuction guiding life decisions" (Knapp et al., 1981, p. 38). Therefore, messages that are received during FC have the potential to act as "rules of conduct" for the survivors regarding their future behavior. Further, the recipient of the message usually participates in constructing parts of the message that are implicit (Knapp et al., 1981). Thereby, the recipient of the FC message should feel empowered because of his or her role in cocreating the message because of his or her inherent understanding of the dying person's intent. Finally, the message can usually be applied to a number of situations, thereby increasing the number of associations and the repetition of the message (Knapp et al., 1981). Sharing messages with others—thereby increasing the redundancy of the message—often increases the memorability of the message (Honeycutt & Cantrill, 2001). Thus, the power and impact of the FC message about religious faith and spirituality would be reiterated every time that it is applied to additional, relevant situations and shared with others. Knapp et al. (1981) stated the following "memorable messages are a rich source of information about our selves, our society, and our ways of communicating" (p. 40). Examination of religious discourse contained in FC from the framework of memorable messages provides a way to explain the profound impact that these end-of-life conversations have on people. Thus, the second research question that this article addresses follows:

RQ2:   What "rules of conduct" pertaining to spirituality or religiosity emerge from FC?

METHOD

Participants and Procedures

Thirty retrospective interviews were conducted in a private office ($N = 30$). The sample consisted of 26 women and 4 men: 24 of the participants were White, 5 were Hispanic, and 1 was Black. Participants ranged in age from 21 to 85, with the average age of the participants being 38. Broad sampling techniques were used to obtain the purposive sample included in this research. Purposive sampling is often necessary in health communication research projects if researchers hope to have an "information rich" sample (Devers & Frankel, 2000). Participants for this study were obtained primarily from a snowball sampling technique (Lindlof, 1995). Participants heard about the research project from other participants, from friends and family members who had heard about the research project through a wide variety of sources, or from the researcher. A flyer was posted in public places and given to hospice programs and grief counselors; a web page was created and sent to a number of different search engines; the researcher talked about the project during one-on-one conversations that were appropriate and gave presentations at meetings. To participate in the study, participants had to meet two criteria: (a) have had a FC or experience (nonverbal interaction) with a loved one, with both participants' knowledge and understanding that one of them was dying; and (b) have a clear recollection of the FC interaction that took place any time between the diagnosis of "terminal amount of time to live" and the actual death.

All participants contacted the researcher about interest in participating to reduce invading people's privacy or pressuring anyone to participate. People in the midst of great pain or emotional stress are often in no shape to participate in an interview (Morse, 2000). Questioning participants about their communication and experiences in the midst of the situation can break down defense mechanisms and bring emotional pain back into focus (Morse, 2000). Conducting interviews in such conditions would be unthinkable and unethical. Under such conditions, utilizing retrospective interviews allows participants to share their insights and their stories under their own terms. Such qualitative methods are appropriate and the best choice to reveal meanings people assign to their personal experiences (Polkinghorne, 1988); to describe the phenomenon through an analysis of the words and nonverbal behaviors; and to create a holistic picture of the phenomenon (Creswell, 1998). Qualitative interview procedures have the potential to reevoke powerful emotional responses (McLeod, 1994), with this study on FC being extremely sensitive and emotional; thus, great care was taken not to pressure or pursue any person to participate.

Only retrospective interviews were conducted, with a simple 10-min focusing exercise used to help participants recall their FC before the actual interview began. Retrospective interviews about major life-altering events such as the death of a loved one often result in a "resurgence of the memories and emotions and brings back experiences" (Morse, 2000, p. 541). Retrospective interviews give people an opportunity to reconstruct their experience and examine perceptions in a new light. This new perspective may be more revealing than it could have been earlier when shrouded in the pain and stress accompanying a loved one's death. Retrospective interviews provide valuable data concerning the "meanings that people ascribe to their own and others' behaviors during communication episodes" (Metts, Sprecher, & Cupach, 1991, p. 164).

The amount of time between the loved one's death and the interview regarding the FC ranged from 3 months to 27 years, with the average amount of time being 6.8 years (two were less than 6 months; seven were 1 to 2 years; nine were 3 to 5 years; three were 5 to 10 years; five were 10 to 15 years; and two were 20 to 27 years). Given the exploratory nature of the study, the interviews were conducted using a semistructured focused format with open-ended questions (Kvale, 1996; McCracken, 1988; Stewart & Cash, 2000). Following an "Emotionalist" perspective, the interviewer formulated open-ended questions that created a climate of rapport which allowed for an honest expression of emotions and "lived experiences" (D. Silverman, 2001). From this perspective, interviewers are encouraged to "become emotionally involved with respondents and to convey their own feelings to both respondents and readers" (D. Silverman, 2001, p. 91). Reason and Rowan (1981) suggested that in-depth interviews in which the interviewee and interviewer become "peers" or "companions" create the possibility of a deep mutual understanding.

The interview guide consisted of 24 open-ended questions with additional questions determined by the flow of the interview. A grief counselor verified the relevance and utility of the interview guide. Interviews lasted between 60 to 120 min, with the average length at approximately 90 min. A six-step process was used during the interview. First, a period of time was taken to make the participant comfortable. Second, participants completed and signed an informed consent. Third, participants completed a brief questionnaire regarding demographic information and the person with whom they had the FC. Fourth, participants completed 10 min of free writing as a focusing exercise concerning their FC. Fifth, the participants were asked a series of interview questions by the investigator primarily in face-to-face interviews (two interviews were conducted via the telephone). Sixth, all participants were debriefed about the interview, their emotional well-being, and their impressions of the experience. Interviews were audiorecorded and transcribed verbatim, resulting in 390 single-spaced pages of data.

Data Analysis

The objective of this type of investigation is to explain recurring patterns of meaning and behaviors of participants (Creswell, 1998; Miles & Huberman, 1984). The researcher utilized both grounded theory and a memorable messages framework to make sense of the participants' experiences. The first goal of the analysis was to describe the meaning of participants' experiences through an examination of recurring patterns (Creswell, 1998; Strauss & Corbin, 1990). The second goal was to approach the data openly but within the framework of memorable messages for additional explanation of the findings (Knapp et. al., 1981).

To gain a holistic understanding of the data, the transcripts were read in their entirety before coding. The process of coding that was used in this research was an adaptation of Glaser and Strauss's (1967) grounded theory (Strauss & Corbin, 1990). For this article, only those messages regarding issues having to do with spirituality, faith, or religion during FC were used. Through open and axial coding, emergent themes and memorable messages were identified (Spradley, 1979; Strauss & Corbin, 1990). Open coding is an iterative process where data are compared for similarity and difference (Strauss & Corbin, 1990). Open coding is also an emergent process where categories are continually added, combined, and revised. Once open coding was completed, axial coding was performed. Axial coding involves making connections between the data that were open coded, a process of searching for commonalities (Strauss & Corbin, 1990). Axial coding involves integrating findings from the different messages to find more general themes that make the analysis coherent. The constant comparative method was used to identify the themes (Strauss & Corbin, 1990). The meanings of the participants' statements were read, reread, and reflected on to identify the important messages for each of the categories.

After the data set was coded, the researcher used the negative case analysis technique to ensure that categories were not forced on the data (Erlandson, Harris, Skipper, & Allen, 1993). A negative case analysis is an interpretive method where data are examined to search for alternative explanations that would render the findings invalid. The researcher continually looked for rival explanations for the research findings (Miles & Huberman, 1998). Once the data was identified, categorized, and coded, the researcher engaged in participant checking (Creswell, 1998; Lincoln & Guba, 1985). Participant checking enabled the researcher the opportunity to see if the interpretation was a valid representation of participants' experiences. Five participants were contacted to discuss the findings, chosen because of the integral role that spirituality or religiosity played in their FC, their representativeness of the population in regard to their FC experiences, and because of their level of competence (e.g., education level or experience with end-of-life issues). Participant checking confirmed the findings that the themes and structures were consistent with their FC experiences in regard to the spiritual or religious faith aspect of their experiences.

RESULTS

Not all participants spoke of issues relating to religion or spirituality during their FC with the dying loved one, but 26 (87%) participants mentioned issues revolving around religious faith or spirituality. One encompassing theme with two distinct subthemes for communication about religious faith or spirituality during FC emerged. These themes provide insights about the form and function of religious faith and spirituality messages during FC. Also, an examination of the data within the theoretical framework of memorable messages revealed three rules of conduct.

Themes of Religious Faith or Spirituality

The overarching theme associated with messages of religious faith or spirituality in FC was validation. All 26 participants validated their (or the dying person's) religious or spiritual beliefs by expressing them during FC. One of the 26 expressed anger at God, but did not feel that her beliefs were invalidated; in fact, she talked about the importance of faith for her family, for the loved one who died, and for herself. In some instances, the reference to faith, religion, or spirituality was very brief, whereas in others it was almost the entire focus of the FC. Validation took three forms: (a) a statement of confirmation of long-held belief systems, (b) a statement of resurrection of dormant belief systems, or (c) a statement of authentication of a perceptual shift in belief. Two functions were served by messages pertaining to survivors' validation of religious or spiritual beliefs: (a) validation and comfort, or (b) validation and community.

Validation and comfort.   Fifteen interviews exemplified the category of validation and comfort, highlighting the solace found when survivors and the dying communicate openly about God's will, a strong belief in an afterlife, or experiences that confirm that there is an afterlife:

> Participant 16: I told my dying son "You know that God is a very powerful part of our lives. I have always tried to teach that to you." And he said, "Yes mom, I know." I said, "So grab a hold of him Jacob. Grab a hold of him and don't let go … Jesus is here to help you … " … And it is so ironic how God had a hand and plans things so well … … "I just want you to know, that you do what you need to do. What God wants you to do."
>
> Participant 30: You can't go through this … witnessing death, without that awe of what life is. Where it comes from and where it goes … (Lines 537–549).

The next example is from an older participant whose life's work as a lawyer was based on fact and rationality. He spent a great deal of time giving background about his mother, father, and himself. He shared a story that his mother told him right before she died. It was about an experience that had happened to her 10 years previously, but she had not told anyone else about the experience, until this FC with her son:

> Participant 29: She said, "He walked out of that door. I know it was him. He came over to me and got me by the arms and lifted me up and he held me in his arms, and he told me, 'I have been permitted to come see you … I'm permitted this one visit.'" And he held her in his arms and he turned and walked away. She felt him, she saw him, she heard him … When she told me that story, I knew that she knew it was true … I'm a rationalist and I'm skeptical. But I knew that she knew that happened. And because she told me it did, I believe it did.

Validation and community.   The idea of "community" at death encompasses participating in the death process to attend to the fate of the dying, and to make the dying easier for the loved ones and others present at the death who are also affected by the death. The results suggest that religious faith and spirituality as discussed during FC led survivors to consider the fragile nature of human life, which led to an appreciation of the significance of community (Heinz, 1999). Eleven people were identified as discussing religious faith or spirituality as part of the validation and community. In addition to messages that authenticated their religious or spiritual beliefs, six of these participants provided examples of how they actively partici- pated in sharing in the death process and in helping their loved one "pass over" through their words or their physical presence:

> Participant 2: He said, "I'm seeing something that I need to tell you." ... "I'm walking up a mountain, and it's um really a beautiful forest and the air smells really pure and clear and white pines ... And I get to the top of the mountain. And there are stars. I've never seen so many stars." And then he said, "All I have to do is step off into the stars and there is God." ... And so then he came back down the mountain and he said that um they had told him that what he should be doing next would be midwifing people who were dying. And that I should be doing it from one side and he would be doing it from the other.

It was very important to the dying husband and the surviving wife that he shared his vision with her, that she believed in the "truth" of his vision, and that she would become a midwife for dying people in the future. Later in the interview, she talked about how she in fact did midwife her young husband through his own death by her actions and her words.

Words suggesting death was not an end and that the two would meet again on another dimension other than earth were representative of community belief in an afterlife:

> Participant 10: ... I was the last one to say goodbye. And I just went over and I just, I took his hand and said, "See you soon. ... I just need you to know that you need to do whatever it is you need to do. And if that's to leave this earth, just know that I'll take care of Ruth."

This participant also talked about a powerful experience that happened to her a short time later that demonstrates the validation and community theme of helping the loved one cross over; as well as the importance of supporting and helping in the midst of grieving:

> Participant 10: I had my eyes closed ... all of a sudden I could see the ceiling in the room I was in, and his light came and just settled in on top of me. And I could feel this spirit in me. Just a part of me. I wasn't scared, you know ... it didn't bother, bother me. I just laid there and I went ... I said, "CC, it's okay. You can go. You can go." ... I could see it [a light or energy] come up above me, and just for a split second, it just hovered there and then it went out the window of the hospital ... within ... about two minutes, three minutes, I

heard 'em call Code Blue. And it was for CC. And he was gone ... You know, we weren't suppose to be there that weekend. And we were. And that's why. We were there so that I could tell CC to go ahead and go on. And it was okay. And support Ruth.

Participant 7: He said, "You don't need to worry about me." He said, "I'm going to heaven ... And that Jesus is my savior, and he is yours too. And you don't ever forget it." ... that was the thing that he wanted us to know most of all (Lines 61–68). ... that was his final and most important opportunity to be a witness to his faith, to his family. And especially to my brother and I.

Rules of Conduct

The form that most religious and spiritual discourse takes during FC is in statements of validation, reflecting comfort or community. The patterns sometimes prescribe behavior, supporting the validity of FC as a type of memorable messages. Three such "Rules of Conduct" were identified as follows: (a) cope with life's challenges after a loved one is gone, (b) be involved in the death and dying process, and (c) enact or live your religion or spirituality.

Cope with life's challenges after their loved one is gone.   The first rule of conduct addresses how the individual should cope with life's challenges after his or her loved one is gone. Eleven of the 26 messages revolving around religious faith or spirituality provide examples of ways that people should face life's challenges. These messages recommend that in times of stress, the individual look to the loved one who has passed because they will be there to help, or reflect on the lessons that were learned in the past (usually taught by the dying person):

Participant 13: "Pray to me. ... And I want you to try to remember what, whatever has happened, instead of looking back on it ... in a way that will make you feel bad, look at [it] as a learning experience. And learn from these things."

Participant 17: When you get to heaven, you know, keep an eye out on my girls. She said, "I will." ... I know I haven't met [the little one], but I love her ... I will, you know, I'll be their guardian angel (Lines 86–89).

Participant 22: In the Hebrew language, there is a word called Mitzvah ... it means good deed ... but it's also interpreted as good deed ... without expecting something in return. And whenever I do those, you know I, I do a good deed or I volunteer. I'm like oh, Dad would have been proud ... that would've made Dad happy ... I'm able to apply [these lessons] all the way, I would hope through the end of my life.

Be involved with the process of death and dying.   The second rule of conduct prescribes how to deal with death and dying. Ten of the 26 messages revolving around religious faith or spirituality that emerged from the data prescribed ways to be involved with the process of death and dying. These messages counseled people not to be afraid but rather to be present and involved with the dying process:

> Participant 10: It's okay to die. It's okay to die. There is a God, or whatever you want to call the higher power. For me it's God. Um, there is a life hereafter. There is a place for us to go. We aren't just living here as a dead end thing, when we die it's over with. Um, but there is a God, or someone smarter than all of us that is directing all of this. And, you know, it took away a lot of that fear of dying. And it just made it dying a part of living, a part of that process … like most families in the United States, we'd never really talked about death and dying. Um, and then, this, this is something that is ongoing in my life now. Where every now and then someone will pop up and I help them die. I will help them say goodbye, help them detach from this earth.
>
> Participant 2: It is important to be kind and present for someone who's dying; if I'm the one who's well and someone else is ill, then it's important for me to be kind and present.
>
> Participant 28: This is as serious as it gets. Don't take it for granted … I knew that who I was and who he was couldn't fit into the mold that society needed us to be in the hush, hush, you know, don't do this. I mean the doctor didn't want me to tell him he was terminal. And my mother-in-law wasn't sure that I should tell him he was terminal. We had to convince her and my father-in-law … I said I can't live a charade with this man. I didn't live a charade with this man when I, when he was home. Why would I do it now? Um it was an eye opener for me, kind of like, "don't leave things unsaid. Don't leave things undone."

Enact or live your religion or spirituality.   The third rule of conduct encourages individuals to enact or live with their religion or spirituality. Five of the 26 messages that emerged from the data revolving around religious faith or spirituality provide examples of prescriptive ways that they live their faith. These messages reflect the importance of being vocal about their faith, to share their beliefs, or the importance of witnessing their faith:

> Participant 6: Death is okay. You know? I mean, I have a strong belief in God. And I felt it that day. And that it's okay to tell people that. … it doesn't need to be in those last hours that it happens.
>
> Participant 7: It's had a big impact on my faith and my spirituality … it's just really made the promise of salvation so real … there wasn't an ounce of

doubt in him … . I've always kept my faith. And it's um, you know … a lot of times people go through periods of doubt and they go off to college and they're, you know, they're free to think the way they want to think. I never really had that.

In sum, the results of this study suggest that discourse about religious faith and spirituality frequently emerge during FCs, with these messages functioning as validation to comfort those left behind and validation to acknowledge death's role as part of the human community. Further, within the memorable messages framework, three lessons associated with rules for living emerged regarding how to cope with life's challenges, deal with death and dying, and enact religion or spirituality in everyday life. The implications for health communicators is far-reaching

DISCUSSION

Although death and communication have been explored for the past 20 to 25 years, it is often done from the dying person's perspective. This article's focus on survivors' perspectives regarding the FC that they had with loved ones before their death begins to fill a gap in the literature associated with death and dying. The participants' reports regarding religious faith and spirituality emerging during FC is consistent with other literature dealing with death, dying, and bereavement (Burck, 1990; Marrone, 1999). When facing death, research has shown that people are often drawn closer to traditional religious beliefs, to beliefs in a caring higher power, to the importance of support from religious or spiritual leaders, to living an ethical life, and to an inner peace in identifying meaning in their lives (Warner, Carment, & Christiana, 1989). People often have a need to transcend death through religious doctrine or new spiritual insights (Marrone, 1999). This research extends these findings by revealing how people communicate about the role of religious faith and spirituality with the dying.

It is commonly believed that experiencing the death of a loved one may challenge people's spiritual or religious beliefs or even invalidate the survivor's faith (Balk, 1999; Marrone, 1999). The findings from this study suggest that communication at the end of life with the loved one may in fact attenuate this outcome and even have the opposite effect for the survivor. Perhaps in the process of talking with a loved one who is dying, survivors come to understand the dying person's religious or spiritual beliefs, experience a spiritual phenomenon during the interaction, or reiterate their own faith in the conversation. This appears to reconfirm beliefs that validate religious faith or spirituality. Thus, the findings in this study suggest that the communication that occurs in the FC is an important factor in validating rather than invalidating the survivor's faith.

The second major theme to emerge in this research, "comforting," in these FC is consistent with previous literature highlighting the importance and role of comforting messages during times of high stress and supportive communication (Burleson, 1994). These messages communicated a high degree of involvement, and were accepting and emotion focused, typical of person-centered comforting messages (Burleson, 1994). Consistent with the outcomes of comforting messages (Burleson, 1994), the validation and comfort messages acknowledged and legitimated both the dying person's and survivor's feelings and beliefs, provided a reduction in the level of distress experienced, and helped the survivor to see how their feelings fit in the broader context of their life. Talking with a dying loved one is a very difficult and emotional interaction, but the participants emphasized how important and comforting it was to have a FC, especially in regard to their spiritual or religious beliefs.

The idea of "community" as revealed in these FC also ties in the idea of a "good" death, which is one in which the dying person is not alone and dies peacefully. There have been "recent writings on 'deathing,' as analogous to 'birthing,' stress [ing] the indispensability of a Lamaze-like coach to the dying—and by extension to the mourner" (Heinz, 1999, p. 165). These FC revealed that a family member or other loved one may be in such a role. They may find themselves unprepared for the event except by reference to religious faith or spirituality as a strategy to assist the dying love one.

Applications and Directions for Future Research

The inadequacy of communication with the dying has often been noted by health caregivers (Thompson & Parrott, 2002). The role of religious faith and spirituality in coping with the inexplicable emerges for family and friends in recalling FC, suggesting that loved ones are unprepared to address these conversations and that death is a time when religious faith and spirituality guide the discourse. These results may be applied to formalize seminars and working groups in organized religious settings for purposes of supporting family members and loved ones of those who have been diagnosed as terminal. As with many issues in health communication, death and dying are stigmatized topics in the larger society, contributing to inadequacy when individuals try to initiate or participate in such conversations. Religious organizations may foster training that health communicators take a role in developing, using findings from this research.

Health care professionals, especially those involved in palliative care, have begun educating the dying about the importance of communicating with loved ones at the end of life. Findings from this study suggest that health care professionals should also educate family members and friends who will endure and survive the death of their loved one about the importance of communicating with the dying person for their benefit. Communication at the end of life can provide validation of one's spiritual or religious beliefs, it can comfort and may lessen the intensity of the grieving experienced by the survivor, and participating as a "witness" to the death may ultimately lessen survivors' own fear of dying. Health communicators may develop messages directed at the general public to generate awareness about the importance and value of participating in FC.

This study sets the stage for larger projects to examine these emergent FC religious or spiritual themes and codes of conduct for their generalizability in larger groups. Additionally, there are a number of directions for future research to take that may address important health and communication outcomes. Two factors to be considered include the following:

1. Can training programs that create awareness about the value and importance of FC decrease the level of fear and apprehension that is associated with talking with people who are dying?
2. Are there health benefits (mental, physical, and emotional) for survivors who engage in FC?

Limitations

This project is based primarily on women, perhaps reflecting a number of gender norms found in the American society. First, most caretakers of terminally ill people are female spouses, mothers, daughters, or daughters-in-law (Davis & Nolen-Hoeksema, 2001). Second, the interviewer is a White woman, and people often feel most comfortable self-disclosing with people who are most similar to them (Gladstein, 1983). Third, men tend to self-disclose intimate and private information with trusted partners and friends rather than strangers (Dindia & Allen, 1992). Fourth, these interviews often elicit a great deal of emotion, and men have been socialized to inhibit emotional displays (Guerrero & Reiter, 1998). The high percentage of White participants may also reflect some cultural bias, as people often prefer to self-disclose to interviewers who are part of their culture (Gladstein, 1983).

A second major limitation revolves around the fact that this is a self-selecting sample. The interviews have primarily portrayed positive FC within primarily positive relationships (two participants did reveal that they had a negative or strained relationship with the dying family member). It is logical to conclude that someone who has had a negative FC would be less likely to volunteer for a project of this nature. Therefore, the experiences of FC that are portrayed may be skewed to a more positive outcome than is representative of society at large.

Ethical Considerations

There are often unforeseeable consequences that come along with writing about people's communication and personal lives (Smythe & Murray, 2000). First, qualitative interview procedures have the potential to reevoke powerful emotional re-sponses (McLeod, 1994). With the FC project, 28 of 30 participants have cried while recalling their private FC with their loved ones (Field notes, October 11, 2002). The interviewer has to be extremely careful, sensitive, and aware of the participants' needs. Second, participants may not be prepared to deal with new feelings or unre-solved conflicts triggered by the questioning (Grafanaki, 1996). Many of the FC pro-ject participants are surprised by the memories that are recalled during the interview process (Field notes, May 14, 2002). Talking out loud for the first time (or for the first time in years) about a sensitive topic such as a FC is bound to generate new insights or emotions that must be dealt with carefully. Third, participants may not be prepared for "the emotional impact of having one's story reinterpreted and filtered through the lenses of social scientific categories" (Smythe & Murray, 2000, p. 321), as it may feel like a cold personification of the person's experience.

CONCLUSIONS

Examining FC has the potential to increase awareness about the importance of communication at the end of life for the survivor. There are messages that can be obtained through FC that may not be revealed at any other time and there are mes-sages that simply reconfirm what is already known. Religious faith or spirituality is an important and, some might say, rather obvious theme of FC. Yet, the role of religious faith and spirituality has been assumed in terms of its service for coping. Rarely has discourse been examined for talk about religious faith and spirituality. Terminality and talk about end of life decision making challenges expert care-givers in health care settings and volunteer caregivers in hospice care programs (see Thompson & Parrott, 2002, for a review). So, it is no small feat to begin to ex-amine the conversations that individuals have about religious faith and spirituality, with a retrospective of these events affording a microcosm in which the lessons learned become memorable guides for the living. These interviews on FC substan-tiate Aiken's (2001) claim that "a consequence of openness toward death is mean-ingful communication with others" (p. 296).

REFERENCES

Aiken, L. R. (2001). *Dying, death, and bereavement* (4th ed.). Mahwah, NJ: Lawrence Erlbaum Associ-ates, Inc.

Balk, D. E. (1999). Bereavement and spiritual change. *Death Studies, 23,* 485–494.

Burck, J. R. (1990). God-talk at the death bed (N1). *Religious Edition, 85,* 557–570.

Burleson, B. R. (1987). Cognitive complexity. In J. C. McCroskey & J. A. Daly (Eds.), *Personality and interpersonal communication* (pp. 305–349). Newbury Park, CA: Sage.

Burleson, B. R. (1994). Comforting messages: Features, functions, and outcomes. In J. A. Daly & J. M. Wiemann (Eds.), *Strategic interpersonal communication* (pp. 135–161). Hillsdale, NJ: Lawrence Erlbaum Associates, Inc.

Callanan, M., & Kelley, P. (1992). *Final gifts: Understanding the special awareness, needs, and communications of the dying.* New York: Bantam.

Creswell, J. W. (1998). *Qualitative inquiry and research design: Choosing among five traditions.* Thousand Oaks, CA: Sage.

Davis, C. G., & Nolen-Hoeksema, S. (2001). How do people make sense of loss? *American Behavioral Scientist, 44*(5), 726–741.

Devers, K. J., & Frankel, R. M. (2000). Study design in qualitative research—2: Sampling and data collection strategies. *Education For Health: Change in Learning and Practice, 13,* 263–272.

Dindia, K., & Allen, M. (1992). Sex differences in self-disclosure: A meta-analysis. *Psychological Bulletin, 112,* 106–124.

Doka, K. J. (1993). *Living with life-threatening illness.* New York: Lexington.

Dull, V. T., & Skokan, L. A. (1995). A cognitive model of religion's influence on health. *Journal of Social Issues, 51*(2), 49–64.

Erlandson, D. A., Harris, E. L., Skipper, B. L., & Allen, S. D. (1993). *Doing naturalistic inquiry: A guide to methods.* Newbury Park, CA: Sage.

Fieweger, M., & Smilowitz, M. (1984). Relational conclusion through interaction with the dying. *Omega, 15,* 61–172.

FitzSimmons, E. (1994). One man's death: His family's ethnography. *Omega, 30,* 23–39.

Gentile M., & Fello, M. (1990). Hospice care for the 1990's. *Journal of Home Health Care Practice, 3,* 1–15.

Gladstein, G. A. (1983). Understanding empathy: Integrating counseling, developmental, and social psychology perspectives. *Journal of Counseling Psychology, 30,* 467–482.

Glaser, B. G, & Strauss, A. L. (1967). *The discovery of grounded theory: Strategies for qualitative research.* New York: Aldine de Gruyter.

Gold, M. (1984). When someone dies in the hospital. *Aging, 345,* 18–22.

Grafanaki, S. (1996). How research can change the researcher: The need for sensitivity, flexibility and ethical boundaries in conducting qualitative research in counseling/psychotherapy. *British Journal of Guidance and Counseling, 24,* 329–338.

Guerrero, L. K., & Reiter, R. L. (1998). Expressing emotion: Sex differences in social skills and communicative responses to anger, sadness, and jealousy. In D. A. Canary & K. Dindia (Eds.), *Sex differences and similarities in communication* (pp. 321–350). Mahwah, NJ: Lawrence Erlbaum Associates, Inc.

Heinz, D. (1999). *The last passage.* New York: Oxford University Press.

Honeycutt, J. M., & Cantrill, J. G. (2001). *Cognition, communication, and romantic relationships.* Mahwah, NJ: Lawrence Erlbaum Associates, Inc.

Knapp, M. L., Stohl, C., & Reardon, K. K. (1981). "Memorable messages." *Journal of Communication, 31*(X), 27–41.

Kubler-Ross, E. (1969). *On death and dying.* New York: Touchstone.

Kvale, S. (1996). *InterViews: An introduction to qualitative research interviewing.* Thousand Oaks, CA: Sage.

Leis, A. M., Kristjanson, L., Koop, P. M., & Laizner, N. (1997). Family health and the palliative care trajectory: A cancer research agenda. *Cancer Prevention and Control, 1,* 352–360.

Lincoln, Y. S., & Guba, E. G. (1985). *Naturalistic inquiry.* Beverly Hills, CA: Sage.

Lindlof, T. R. (1995). *Qualitative communication research methods.* Thousand Oaks, CA: Sage.

Lynn, J., Harrold, J., & The Center To Improve Care of the Dying. (1999). *Handbook for mortals.* New York: Oxford University Press.

Marrone, R. (1999). Dying, mourning, and spirituality: A psychological perspective. *Death Studies, 23,* 495–519.

Marshall, V. W. (1975). Socialization for impending death in a retirement village. *American Journal of Sociology, 80,* 1124–1144.

McCracken, G. (1988). *The long interview.* Newbury Park, CA: Sage.

McGrath, P. A., Yates, P., Clinton, M., & Hart, G. (1999). "What should I say?": Qualitative findings on dilemmas in palliative care nursing. *Hospice Journal, 14,* 17–33.

McKenzie, S. C. (1980). *Aging and old age.* Glenview, IL: Scott, Foresman.

McLeod, J. (1994). *Doing counseling research.* London: Sage.

Metts, S., Sprecher, S., & Cupach, W. R. (1991). Retrospective self-reports. In B. M. Montgomery & S. Duck (Eds.), *Studying interpersonal interaction* (pp. 162–178). New York: Guilford.

Miles, M. B., & Huberman, A. M. (1984). *Qualitative data analysis* (2nd ed.). Thousand Oaks, CA: Sage.

Morse, J. M. (2000). Researching illness and injury: Methodological considerations. *Qualitative Health Research, 10,* 538–546.

Nadeau, J. W. (1998). *Families making sense of death.* Thousand Oaks, CA: Sage

Nolen-Hoeksema, S., & Larson, J. (1999). *Coping with loss.* Mahwah, NJ: Lawrence Erlbaum Associates, Inc.

Nussbaum, J. F., Pecchioni, L. L., Robinson, J. D., & Thompson, T. L. (2000). *Communication and aging* (2nd ed.). Mahwah, NJ: Lawrence Erlbaum Associates, Inc.

Pargament, K. I. (1999). The psychology of religion and spirituality? Yes and no. *International Journal for the Psychology of Religion, 9,* 3–16.

Polkinghorne, D. E. (1988). *Narrative knowing and the human sciences.* Albany: State University of New York Press.

Reason, P., & Rowan, J. (1981). *Human inquiry.* New York: Wiley.

Silverman, D. (2001). *Interpreting qualitative data: Methods of analysing talk, text, and interaction* (2nd ed.). Thousand Oaks, CA: Sage.

Silverman, P. R., Weiner, A., & El Ad, N. (1995). Parent–child communication in bereaved Israeli families. *Omega, 3,* 217–225.

Smythe, W. E., & Murray, M. J. (2000). Owning the story: Ethical considerations in narrative research. *Ethics & Behavior, 10,* 311–336.

Spradley, J. P. (1979). *The ethnographic interview.* New York: Holt, Rinehart and Winston.

Stewart, C. J., & Cash, W. B. (2000). *Interviewing: Principles and practices* (9th ed.). Boston: McGraw-Hill.

Strauss, A., & Corbin, J. (1990). *Basics of qualitative research: Grounded theory procedures and techniques.* Newbury Park, CA: Sage.

Thompson, T. L., & Parrott, R. (2002). Interpersonal communication and health care. In M. L. Knapp & J. A. Daly (Eds.), *Handbook of interpersonal communication* (pp. 680–725). Thousand Oaks, CA: Sage.

Underwood, L. G., & Teresi, J. A. (2002). The daily spiritual experience scale: Development, theoretical description, reliability, exploratory factor analysis, and preliminary construct validity using health-related data. *Annals of Behavioral Medicine, 24,* 22–33.

Warner, R., Carment, G., & Christiana, N. M. (1989). The spiritual needs of persons with AIDS. *Family and Community Health, 12,* 43–51.

HEALTH COMMUNICATION, *16*(1), 105–116

Talking About Human Genetics Within Religious Frameworks

Tina M. Harris
Department of Speech Communication
University of Georgia

Roxanne Parrott
Department of Communication Arts & Sciences
The Pennsylvania State University

Kelly A. Dorgan
Department of Communication
East Tennessee State University

Information generated by the Human Genome Project is intended to result in better understanding of genetic variation and disease, affording opportunities to intervene in human health both prior to and after birth. The lay public's construction of meaning associated with these aims, however, has been given little systematic consideration. As God and religion are often invoked as structures to give meaning to technical and scientific discoveries, this project sought to examine public discussions associated with religious frameworks used to talk about human genetics. The results of 17 focus group discussions revealed a range of lay epistemologies that suggest how religious faith may impact individual perceptions, with some consistent differences in discourse for African Americans as compared to European Americans observed. The ethical and practical applications of this information are extended to suggestions for health promotion, care, and counseling.

Information generated by the Human Genome Project (HGP) is intended to result in better understanding of genetic variation and disease, affording opportunities to intervene in human health both prior to and after birth (Mahowald, Levinson, &

Requests for reprints should be sent to Tina M. Harris, 128 Terrell Hall, Department of Speech Communication, University of Georgia, Athens, GA 30602. E-mail: tmharris@arches.uga.edu

Cassel, 1996; Oktay, 1998). Based on historical precedence associated with Hitler and efforts to design a "master race," however, some individuals who have experienced illness or behavior linked to genetics have also expressed concern that the new genetics might be linked to an old aim—to systematically eliminate human "defects" (Kerr, Cunningham-Burley, & Amos, 1998), code for racial or ethnic cleansing (Condit, 1999). This concern may be particularly salient for African Americans (AAs) who live with the legacy of the Tuskegee experiments in which AA men were used in medical research without their informed consent, contributing to mistrust of the American medical system and perhaps greater reliance on religious frameworks to make attributions about health (Cole-Turner, 1999). This research conducted focus groups in the United States to explore AA and European American (EA) lay discourse about human genetics, attending to references with religious or spiritual content.

CONSTRUCTING MEANING ABOUT
GENES AND HEALTH

Humans' spiritual identities and religious faith are central to day-to-day functioning (Getz, 1984), often providing guidelines for living (Clark & Dawson, 1996; Getz, 1984). Lay audiences from various racial backgrounds may invoke religious frameworks to talk about intentions associated with human genetics and the HGP. One study conducted with 20 focus groups in central Scotland, for example, revealed the importance of the expression "drawing the line" in discussions about moral and ethical concerns regarding human genetics research (Kerr et al., 1998). Such expressions afford insights about how lay audiences construct meaning about genetics and health. Based on these insights, health promotion, care, and counseling messages may attempt to accommodate, assimilate, or repattern these beliefs in efforts to acknowledge lay attitudes.

Recognizing the role that religious counselors may play in translating knowledge about genetics and humanity in an age of genomics, Cole-Turner (1999) asserted that, "Ideally, genetic counselors and clergy should be in communication with each other and should work together in a way that complements each other's work" (p. 208). This principle for practice acknowledges the importance of religious frameworks in decision making around genes and health; yet, it largely ignores the reality that lay audiences construct meaning about genes and health based on understanding derived from both of these two expert realms. Individuals who are not experts in either genetic counseling or religion make decisions about genes and health based on the meanings they construct from both realms. In turn, the ways that lay audiences talk about genes and health within religious frameworks may reflect such understanding.

Religious orientation is central to a person's attitude toward health (Forthun, Bell, Peek, & Sun, 1999). Differences in religious orientations have been observed between AAs and EAs that may impact the acceptance of human genome research (e.g., Chatters & Taylor, 1998) and be revealed in the discourse of each group talking about a role for religious faith in human genetics. AAs, who have high religiosity (Carlton-LaNey, Hamilton, Ruiz, & Alexander, 2001) and rely on religious faith to deal with various circumstances (Taylor, Chatters, Jayakody, & Levin, 1996), tend to report high levels of public (e.g., religious attendance) and private (e.g., reading religious materials) religious behaviors, engaging in daily prayer and believing that the Bible is the Word of God (Musgrove, Allen, & Allen, 2002). AAs often personalize their relationship with God, even forming expectations around God as a "health communicator" who "provides information through various mechanisms" that include prophesies and dreams foretelling future health events (McCauley, Pecchioni, & Grant, 2000, p. 25). The discourse that AAs use in talking about the role of God in genes and health may thus differ from that used by EAs. An examination of discursive practices from both groups provides the only means, however, to ascertain whether such differences exist.

Health communicators have applied research that reveals the importance of religious activities for AAs as evidence to support the efficacy of delivering health promotion efforts targeting AAs via community-based church settings (e.g., Resnicow et al., 2001). The research associating AA's religiosity with health attitudes and behaviors has not, however, contributed to efforts to incorporate these beliefs and attitudes, including the discursive expressions associated with religion and health, into counseling, care, or promotion messages. This may be due to an absence of knowledge associated with such discursive practice and instead reliance on sites such as churches and sources such as ministers as a strategy to reach those who are religious with health messages. This is, of course, an important venue for the application of previous research but only a first step, as religious faith comprises a worldview that may shape responses to health messages. Thus, the delivery of traditional health education and information through nontraditional sites and sources ignores the need to tailor health messages to religiosity.

Discursive practices associated with genes and health may include expressions associated with the belief that disease is God's punishment for a personal wrong or sin, or illness is a life lesson (Weil, 1991). One study that examined perceptions about causes of a birth defect or genetic disorder, for example, found that AAs believed that God punished parents by causing a child to have a birth defect more often than EAs or Hispanics did (Cohen, Fine, & Pergament, 1998). Whether they talk about health conditions in this way, however, is another matter. Health care, counseling, and promotions messages may have little impact for those who hold such beliefs if messages fail to include references that reflect the ways that they talk about the issues. Health communicators are increasingly aware of the necessity of broadly defining health literacy, encompassing cultural differences associated with how health values are described, and talk about personal control over health. For example, a study of 111 mothers of children with a genetic disorder found that those who least believed in the role of environmental factors (e.g., radiation, accident, or injury) or personal behaviors (e.g., medication, alcohol, or drug use) on such disease were most likely to believe that "God causes it," or "I was chosen" (Weil, 1991). Again, how such beliefs are reflected in the ways that genes and health are discussed by lay audiences are not known. Others have asserted that one avenue for health communicators to bridge gaps between science and religion is greater understanding of how lay audiences talk about religious faith and its role in health (Valenti, 2002). Toward that aim and efforts to guide the communication of genetic information to the lay public, this research examined the following:

RQ1:   How do lay audiences describe God's role in health and human genes?
RQ2:   Do these descriptions differ between AAs as compared to EAs?

METHOD

Participants

During the Winter and Spring of 2000, 17 focus groups (5 EA men, 4 EA women, 5 AA women, and 4 AA men) were conducted as part of the formative evaluation phase for a project examining the lay public's understanding of human genetics. Participants ($N = 82$) included 39 women (including 19 AAs) and 43 men (including 23 EAs), with 81% indicating they had medical insurance. The average age of participants was 28.55 years ($SD = 6.19$). Income ranged from 16% who made less than $10,000, 24% in the $10,000 to $25,000 range, 29% making $25,000 to $40,000, 10% in the $40,000 to $55,000 range, and 16% making $55,000 or more. Nearly half had some college, with 46.3% indicating they had completed a college course in biology.

Procedures

Several methods were used to recruit participants, including telephone solicitation via random digit dialing ($n = 29$), trained community sponsorship ($n = 34$), and a snowball technique ($n = 19$) in which individuals informed and then recruited acquaintances to participate in the project. The community sponsors were recruited from area organizations (beauty and barber shops, and a local computer company) via the researchers, provided with a project overview, and asked to recruit participants. Two questions were asked to screen all potential participants: (a) Have you ever had a genetic test or received genetic counseling and (b) how much do you know about human genetics, with responses ranging from "*know nothing at all*" to "*know all that there is to know."* Individuals who had received genetic testing or counseling, or answered that they "know all there is to know" or "know a great deal" about human genetics were eliminated from further consideration for participation as a method of defining the "lay" as compared to a more knowledgeable or experienced public. Participants received a reminder telephone call the night before a scheduled meeting, a parking voucher, a $50 honorarium, and a light meal during the meeting. Transportation following the meetings was available, as was child care during the meetings. The meetings lasted between 90 min and 2 hr. Recruitment proceeded until an approximately equal number of AA and EA men and women had participated.

Focus group meetings were held in a southeastern town associated with a large land grant institution. When participants arrived for the focus group, they were greeted and asked to fill out a brief sociodemographic form that included a request for age, gender, race, and income. Participants were not asked for specific religious affiliations but were asked to indicate the following: "In describing yourself, how religious are you?" Nine participants chose not to answer, including 6 AA women, 2 AA men, and 1 EA men. Eighteen participants said that they were very religious (60% AA), 37 indicated that they were somewhat religious (46% EA), 12 were not religious, 3 were somewhat negative, and 3 EAs were very negative toward religion. Trained moderators were of the same race as participants in the focus groups to increase comfort levels for disclosing about issues that have historical racial parameters. The focus groups were video and audio recorded. Complete transcripts of the focus group discussions were produced, with a professional transcriber's work followed by the moderator of the group reviewing the document with the audio and, if necessary, video recording to fill in any missing information.

During the focus groups, participants addressed questions and probes associated with the lay public's understanding of genes and health. This study analyzes focus group discussions that centered on the question, "How does God relate to genes?" and the follow-ups: (a) "Does God work through genes? In other words, is God the Creator of our genes? Can God change our genes before we are born? Can God change our genes after we are born? How might that happen?" and (b) "Does God work independently of genes? In other words, if we have a gene linked to disease, can God affect whether we get the disease? How might that happen?" References to God or religious faith made before or after the specific question were included in the analysis as well.

Data Analysis

Three techniques were employed to establish trustworthiness in the blended manifest and latent content analysis, as recommended for coding data such as transcripts and field notes (Berg, 1998). First, a qualitative latent analysis was used, with three coders independently reading the transcripts (Lincoln & Guba, 1985), and using the talk turn as the unit of analysis to highlight any references with spiritual or religious connotations. This open coding promoted the likelihood that all references to God and religion would be noted. A textual search of such terms as "He" in reference to God, for example, would have overreached references to God's role. Failure to identify instances where references were made to a deity in terms other than "God," however, would have underestimated such references.

The results of the initial coding were reviewed and discussed, leading to the identification of several consistent phrases or ways of talking about the role of God in genes and health. The transcripts were coded independently a second time with these in mind to identify any additional references. As part of this manifest content analysis, a text search was performed using QSR NUD*IST to identify and provide countable themes in the transcripts in association with references to "God" and the codes used during the latent content analysis, promoting a more complete analysis of the data (Berg, 1998), and a check on the latent analysis (Babbie, 1998). QSR Nudist (Non-numerical Unstructured Data Indexing Searching and Theorizing) software is a program that is exclusively used for the analysis of qualitative data. Use of this program allows qualitative researchers to make sense of complex data. In general, text transcripts from focus groups and other forms of qualitative data are auto coded, which allows researchers to discover or locate patterns or themes that naturally emerge from the data. To reflect the manifest analysis, some quantitative data are presented throughout the Results section. Findings are supported by at least three examples for each assertion (Babbie, 1998; Berg, 1998).

RESULTS

The results revealed that 73 of the 82 focus group participants took part in the discussion about God, religious faith, spirituality, and genes, with 261 talk turns devoted to discussion of this subject. The EA female groups had 96 such turns, ranging from 11 to 31 units in a single group, and all EA women participated. Among the 5 AA female focus groups, there were 37 talk turns devoted to the topic, ranging between 5 and 10 turns within a group; in 3 groups, all members participated; one member in each of the other 2 groups did not directly discuss religion. Fewer in number than talk turns in the EA female groups, turns were often longer as the women elaborated on their views. In the EA male groups, 63 talk turns addressed the focal topic, ranging between 11 and 25, with all members participating in this discussion in 2 groups, whereas 2 other groups had some members who did not participate. In the AA male groups, 65 turns were devoted to the topic with all participants involved in 2 groups whereas the other 2 groups did not have all members engaging in discussion; the number of turns ranged between 14 and 19. Four of the 5 AA women's groups raised the topic of God and genes before the moderator raised it as a direct topic for discussion, as did 1 AA male group and 1 EA female group. Excerpts to illustrate participant comments are referred to by their assigned participant and focus group numbers. For example, Participant 62 (European American woman) would be identified with (EAW62:FG3) at the end of her statement.

Uncertainty About God's Role

Several participants indicated that they were uncertain about the role a higher power might play in human genetics. As one participant simply stated, "I have no idea" (EAW60:FG2). A total of seven participants noted that although the focus group discussion about "God's role" in genetics started them thinking about the matter, they had previously never thought about the issue. As one EA female focus group member stated, "I don't know what I think," suggesting either an inability or unwillingness to grapple with a potentially unanswerable question (EAW90:FG4). Another participant said, "I'm not sure. I don't know. I'm just not sure" (EAW54:FG1), with a participant in a third EA female group saying, "I don't really have an opinion about God one way or the other" (EAW80:FG3). Some participants directly stated that humans form different belief systems ($n =$ 18), with more direct statements such as, "different people have different ideas about God" (EAW52:FG1), to more indirect statements that included, "You are making the assumption that there is a God which I may not assume" (EAW58:FG1). A small number of participants ($n = 3$) noted that some people have no belief in God. One participant said, "I'm atheist" (EAM65:FG4). Uncertainty was only openly expressed by EAs.

God Made Our Genes

Many AA and EA participants across the 17 groups conveyed the conviction that God created genes, affirming belief in a higher power's role in human creation. One half of all participants ($n = 41$) explicitly noted that God "made" human genes. This included 7 EA men, 12 AA men, 9 EA women, and 13 AA women. One participant contended that, "God has the primary role because He is the Creator," adding, "He determines how each one of us will be" (AAW8:FG1). In another focus group, a participant declared, "He created them [genes]. That's my personal belief and I'm not afraid to say it" (EAM59:FG2). In a separate focus group, a member offered, "He created genes. That's what I believe" (EAM93:FG5).

God Does Not Micromanage

Although a sizable number of participants communicated their belief that God created human genes, many EA participants expressed the view that God's role ends at creation. The phrase "humans' free will" appeared 22 times during discussions about the role of God in genes. Some pointed to humans' free will, implicitly overriding a role for God. Others were more direct, with 1 male group member who re-marked, "I think God rolled the dice 19 billion years ago" and then left humanity to its struggle (EAM73:FG4). In a second group, another participant indicated his be-lief that God simply "sets everything into motion" (EAW52:FG1). A third partici-pant said although there may be a "plan at a beginning point," she does not "think that God micromanages" (EAW58:FG1). These participants' words help explain views ($n = 15$) that God plays no ongoing role in human genetics, which emerged only in the EA focus groups.

God Works Through Our Genes

Both genders and races testified to God's divine ability to play an active role in hu-man genetics after birth. Although only EAs expressed a belief that God's role ends at the point of making human genes, 26 participants, both men and women, AA and EA, contended that God could change a person's genes. There was wide variance, however, in the expressions about how or why God would intervene. Some participants' discourse reflected devout faith with little elaboration. One woman stated that, "the Lord can do anything," including play a role in human ge-netics (AAW36:FG2). One man pointed out regarding God's ability to actually change a human's genes, "In God, all things are possible" (AAM21:FG3). Another stated, God "works through genes" (AAM3:FG1). Still another said that God can "heal you" (AAM31:FG4). AA men asserted the possibility for good and bad out-comes associated with divine intervention:

> I hear a lot of people say that after they have had a terrible illness … that they have a deeper appreciation for God, and maybe that's one way God works through genes, as in striking you with that illness. That would be a way to bring you closer to God. (AAM7:FG1)

A theme that repeatedly arose was that human genetics is the domain of God, not humans, and therefore could only be altered by God. For example, God could enact "vengeance" by changing human genes in a negative way, as claimed by 5 AA men. Further, several participants worried that by conducting genetics research, humans are "playing God," or as stated by 1 AA man, "messin' with God" (AAM11:FG2). An EA male participant questioned whether cloning a human is the "right thing to do," suggesting that such behavior may be part of, "Trying to play God" (EAM91:FG5). Another seemed to fear that geneticists are "making changes to something that you are not supposed to be bothering." He warned, "they're taking God's job. That's dangerous. They're trying to do God's work" (AAM21:FG3). One participant pointed to past "human behavior," especially "Adolf Hitler and his Aryan race:" You are going to get people who are going to take it to that extreme because I mean that. He is not the only one who has done it or other people who feel that way. So if you have the ability to develop people, you know, that you consider to be superior over other people … . There are those who are going to use that type of information and power with … to oppress other people (AAW22:FG5)

Humans May Appeal to God

Healing "comes with faith" (AAM21: FG3). Likewise, healing may only come through obedience and adherence to God's laws. As 1 man claimed, if people would simply abide by the Ten Commandments, "Then the world would be a better place and a healthier place" and would "contribute to healthier genes" (AAM7: FG1). The following participant's words potentially reflect the struggle in which some engaged in figuring out God's role:

> Like somebody who had cancer and then boom, and all of a sudden it was gone … I don't know if that would be changing genes or you know … just getting rid of … of the cancer (EAW60: FG2).

As noted by a few participants ($n = 5$), prayer may bring a miracle of healing through God's grace:

> God has always been able to work miracles. So if you had a problem with a gene or a disease or if you had a genetic—If you prayed about it and if you had faith that you weren't going to get it, I believe that God is able to change that. (AAW38: FG2)

In another focus group, a participant linked the notion of free will to miracles, saying that although God "allows us to make our own choices" that "He can intervene through grace" (AAW22: FG5). The latter example provides a conditional part of such belief. If a person has faith and prays, God may change the effects of genes as part of His ultimate plan. As 1 woman stated, "God has always been able to work miracles." She continued, "if you prayed about it and if you had faith that you weren't going to get it, I believe that God is able to change that" (AAW38: FG2). Similarly, some participants communicated that God may also choose not to change the effects. That "He" may be "challenging" a person and building character. For example, 1 woman pointed out that "if you were pregnant and you find the child had some kind of illness or whatever, how strong is your faith? God gave you that child" (AAW4: FG1).

DISCUSSION

Scholarly inquiry focused on how lay audiences' talk about religious faith and genetics may aid health communicators in providing culturally sensitive guidelines that contribute to effective health promotion, care, and counseling. Talk about God's role in human genetics revealed through the conversations of focus group participants in this research illustrated an age-old human dilemma, the tension between belief in God's omniscience and humans' free will. Some participants expressed the view that God "determines who we are," and many stated that "God made our genes." Although care must be exercised, this research affords insights about health care, counseling, and promotion efforts associated with genetic information and the lay public.

One goal of genetic research is to offer a variety of advancements that will benefit most, if not all, members of society. Given the history of race and medicine in the United States, however, there are various racial and ethnic group members (e.g., AAs and the Tuskegee Experiment) who have a high level of mistrust for health and science institutions. The fear of being unwilling participants in such research is bolstered by reference to the religious belief that scientists are "playing God." Although AAs have historical basis for their mistrust, EAs, too, fear that human genetic research and genetic technologies are being used inappropriately. This concern must be addressed directly in communication before those for whom such beliefs are a barrier to performance of practices associated with genomic health care are likely to avail themselves of such consultation. Also, there is an evident tension between believing that the possibility of divine intervention exists and believing that it is likely, a tension expressed by one participant's proclamation that she does not believe that "God micromanages." For the unformed attitude group, exposure to appeals aimed at involving individuals concerned that science has gone too far with research in human genetics may shape support for genomics.

One group of individuals in this study did not believe in God. Clearly, such a group exists in the larger society, believing that God and genetic research are not related and should be treated as separate entities. It is not known whether direct appeals interpersonally or through the media that make reference to God would be offensive. Religious faith is a strongly held value. In a nation founded on religious freedom and among citizens who largely claim to be religious, openly declaring one's own lack of religious faith is not a declaration likely to be done with little thought behind it. Thus, appeals from health care providers, genetic counselors, or health promoters that are designed to address God's role in human genes may offend nonbelievers. Any effort to encompass religious faith in the pursuit of strategic communication should be reviewed for insights about ways to limit nonbelievers' feelings of exclusion or even hostility.

Ethical Considerations

One ethical dilemma that has been named by Guttman (1997) as the persuasion dilemma emphasizes the reality that experts in communication use strategies to achieve particular aims that may actually limit an audience's careful consideration of an action. Linking God and religious faith to the promotion of a behavior may or may not produce such passive message processing, but it is a concern that should be systematically examined. Findings such as those in this project, however, suggest that continued neglect of this area in communication studies presents an ethical dilemma of its own.

Limitations

Although the importance of religious faith was supported in this research, there may be great reticence to express a lack of such faith. Only EA participants identified themselves as being negatively predisposed toward religion in this study. Although the question about religion and the responses were confidential, the forum of a focus group makes responses public to the members of the group. A larger sample of individuals with negative attitudes toward religion and a willingness to express them in public discussions may have contributed to different results. Thus, strategic efforts to include religious faith and spirituality in health communication activities must be designed with both believers and nonbelievers in mind, and with no intention to change individual predisposition in this regard.

Directions for Future Research

Strategic efforts should be made to acknowledge and respect the beliefs of individuals who believe that genetic technology is beyond the appropriate realm for humans to play a role. Here is an example of a possible message from health care practitioners that acknowledges religious beliefs while promoting understanding of human genetic research: "From God's vantage point, humans have reached a new frontier—a place where genetic technology may prevent disease. God's waiting for you to do your part. Talk with a health care provider today and see if genetic testing is an appropriate option for you." Similarly, a faith leader, pastor, or minister may state from the pulpit, … "If God is your guide, your prayers that 'God's will be done' together with your requests for 'divine intervention and a healing' may be answered with guidance to seek genetic counseling. Will your heart be listening?" These messages are a far different path than any examined before within the study of social influence. Also, the sources of the lay public's knowledge about genes and health in the religious domain, religious and spiritual leaders, should be consulted for insights about their attitudes and communication with laity about this topic. Together with an examination of actual sermons to assess references to the human genome project, genetics, reproductive technologies, and other related issues, more insightful ways to communicate about the role religious faith in lay attitudes about genes and health may be gained.

ACKNOWLEDGMENT

This research was supported by Grant RO6/CCR319514–02 from the Centers for Disease Control and Prevention to the second author.

REFERENCES

Babbie, E. (1998). *The practice of social research.* Belmont, CA: Wadsworth.

Berg, B. (1998). *Qualitative research methods for the social sciences.* Boston: Allyn & Bacon.

Bourjolly, J. N. (1998). Differences in religiousness among Black and White women with breast cancer. *Social Work in Health Care, 28,* 21–39.

Carlton-LaNey, I., Hamilton, J., Ruiz, D., & Alexander, S. C. (2001). "Sitting with the sick": African American women's philanthropy. *Affilia, 16,* 447–466.

Chatters, L. M., & Taylor, R. J. (1998). Religious involvement among African Americans. *African American Research Perspectives, 4,* 83–93.

Clark, J. W., & Dawson, L. E. (1996). Personal religiousness and ethical judgements: An empirical analysis. *Journal of Business Ethics, 15,* 359–370.

Cohen, L. H., Fine, B. A., & Pergament, E. (1998). An assessment of ethnocultural beliefs regarding the causes of birth defects and genetic disorders. *Journal of Genetic Counseling, 7,* 15–29.

Cole-Turner, R. (1999). Faith meets the human genome project: Religious factors in the public response to genetics. *Public Understanding of Science, 8,* 207–214.

Condit, C. M. (1999). *The meanings of the gene: Public debates about human heredity.* Madison: The University of Wisconsin Press.

Dossey, L. (1993). *Healing words: The power of prayer and the practice of medicine.* New York: Harper.

Forthun, L. F., Bell, N. J., Peek, C. W., & Sun, S. W. (1999). Religiosity, sensation seeking, and alcohol/drug use in denominational and gender contexts. *Journal of Drug Issues, 29,* 75–90.

Getz, I. (1984). The relation of moral reasoning and religion: A review of the literature. *Counseling and Values, 28,* 94–116.

Guttman, N. (1997). Ethical dilemmas in health campaigns. *Health Communication, 9,* 155–190.

Kerr, A., Cunningham-Burley, S., & Amos, A. (1998). Drawing the line: An analysis of lay people's discussions about the new genetics. *Public Understanding of Science, 7,* 113–133.

Lincoln, Y. S., & Guba, E. G. (1985). *Naturalistic Inquiry.* Newbury Park, CA: Sage.

Mahowald, M. B., Levinson, D., & Cassel, C. (1996). The new genetics and women. *Milbank Quarterly, 14,* 239–283.

McAuley, W. J., Pecchioni, L. L., & Grant, J. A. (2002). The impact of living in a rural county with no nursing home on utilization rates and admission mobility patterns. *Journal of Applied Gerontology, 27,* 40–57.

Musgrove, C. F., Allen, C. E., & Allen, G. J. (2002). Spirituality and health for women of color. *American Journal of Public Health, 92,* 557–560.

Oktay, J. S. (1998). Genetics cultural lag: What can social workers do to help? *Health & Social Work, 23,* 310–315.

Resnicow, K., Jackson, A., Wang, T., De., A. K., McCarty, F., Dudley, W. N., et al. (2001). A motivational interviewing intervention to increase fruit and vegetable intake through Black churches: Results of the eat for life trial. *American Journal of Public Health, 91,* 1686–1694.

Taylor, R. J., Chatters, L. M., Jayakody, R., & Levin, J. (1996). Black and White differences in religious participation: A multisample comparison. *Journal for the Scientific Study of Religion, 25,* 403–410.

Valenti, J. M. (2002). Critiques and contentions: Communication challenges for science and religion. *Public Understanding of Science, 11,* 57–63.

Weil, J. (1991). Mothers' postcounseling beliefs about the causes of their children's genetic disorders. *American Journal of Human Genetics, 48,* 145–153.

The Delivery of Health Care in Faith-Based Organizations: Parish Nurses as Promoters of Health

Carolyn M. Anderson

The University of Akron

This research report examines the role of faith-based organizations in the delivery of health care. Special emphasis is given to parish nurse programs and the unique relationship between parish nurses and faith members. Parish nurses attend not only to the physical needs of faith members, but also to needs associated with emotional and spiritual wellness. Parish nurses ($N = 25$) responded to questions about health ministries in faith-based organizations, their role as nurses, and the benefits of partnering with these organizations to promote health care. The nurses described the delivery of care through educational clinics, viewed themselves as promoters of health, and described the benefits of a holistic approach to health that includes emotional and spiritual dimensions. The discussion addresses themes that emerged from the results as well the ethical implications of incorporating health ministries into faith-based organizations.

Many faith-based organizations are mobilizing to deliver health services in a diverse number of communities. The concept of ministering to the sick in places of worship is not new. Before modern medicine and the rise of technology, church members tended the sick, used faith in a divine healer (i.e., God) for emotional support, and participated in public communal prayers for the physical, emotional, and spiritual needs of members (du Pre, 2000). Faith-based organizations are taking steps to reestablish the mission of ministering to the health needs of faith members. One innovative step to accomplish this mission is the establishment of parish nurse programs, health ministries that use registered professional nurses to deliver care to members of faith-based organizations (Solari-Twadell, 1999). Health communication theory and practice may be enriched by an exploration and understanding of this movement. Investigating parish nurse programs may reveal important insights about caregiver

Requests for reprints should be sent to Carolyn M. Anderson, School of Communication, The University of Akron, Akron, OH 44325-1003. E-mail: canders@uakron.edu roles that increase the efficacy of care within formal health systems (Ludwig-Beymer & Sarran, 1999). Parish nurse programs can provide insight for physicians and researchers alike into the process of organizing health care delivery at the community level, as community groups like faith-based organizations often provide a forum for identifying pertinent health problems and at-risk groups in their communities (Solari-Twadell, 1999). Other health care providers and caregivers may gain insights about resources available to many of their patients outside the realm of the formal health care delivery system and strategies to support patients' spiritual needs (Kirschner, 1999). To build a foundation for health communication interest, the following research report examines the role of faith-based organizations in delivering health care and promotion, with a specific focus on parish nurse programs.

AN OVERVIEW OF ORGANIZED HEALTH PROMOTION
AND CARE IN FAITH-BASED SETTINGS

Spirituality is a complex construct. Some view it as an "inner life force or vitality" and others see it as "a connection with an imagined or real power source outside of the natural world" (Lawrence, 2002. p. 74). In ancient times, medical spiritualism was the belief that supernatural forces such as gods or spirits govern over illnesses (Bille, 1981). Relatedly, members of the Christian faith believe that Jesus of Nazareth performed miracles such as healing the physically sick or mentally ill (Carson, 1989; Wylie, 1990). The belief that Jesus performed miracles demonstrates the existence of a personal God who restores health as a reward to believers. Recent trends linking "religion, spirituality, and health" can be traced to two primary issues (Sloan & Bagiella, 2002, p. 14). First, patients are seeking alternatives to the conventional biomedical model of care that has rested on the premise that ill health can be explained and treated with physical means. Engle (1977) explained that a broadened view of the traditional medical model, a biopsychosocial approach, takes into account a person's physical condition, as well as beliefs, values, and social expectations. A second issue contributing to the attention being paid to religion and health is that some research studies have made claims about the positive health effects on illnesses when patients have spiritual involvement in their lives, whereas the opposite is true for those who do not have such involvement (Sloan & Bagiella, 2002).

Arguments in support of the role of faith-based organizations as natural places for dissemination of health information and promotion are rooted in the philosophy that health is more than physical, with a unique interrelation existing between spirituality and health. People who are healthy tend to embrace a holistic view of health that includes spiritual and emotional dimensions (Schnorr, 1999). The following discussion reviews how faith-based organizations are forming health ministries to advance a holistic view of health.

Health Ministries

Health ministries operate within faith-based settings to promote health, including access to health care. Health ministries are organized to include a committee comprised of community members who represent clergy, nurses, physicians, social workers, and laity who may or may not have health or religious expertise and training. The ministries promote the concept of health as the interrelation of body, mind, and spirit. Health ministers will be individuals who are comfortable with prayer and who challenge, enable, nurture, and sustain people to be good stewards of the gift of life (Health Ministries Association, Inc., 2001).

One goal of health ministries is to understand how the relation between health ministers and faith members influences the physical, emotional, and spiritual aspect of faith members' lives (Solari-Twadell, 1999). Health ministers connect with faith members through community involvement and provide social support to faith members in that role. However, health ministers also act as educators, counselors, resource persons, and prayer partners. They are in a position that can promote healthy lifestyles, encourage prevention measures, and embrace the interdependent relation between health and worship. To meet these objectives, many faith-based organizations are establishing parish nurse programs.

Parish Nurse Programs

A parish nurse program is "health ministry using a registered professional nurse" (Solari-Twadell, 1999, p. 3). The idea of nurses working in parishes developed from the work of Granger Westberg, a Lutheran minister and professor at the University of Illinois School of Medicine and Divinity School, together with officials from Lutheran General Hospital located on the outskirts of Chicago. As early as the 1960s and 1970s, they worked with physicians, nurses, clergy, and faith communities to establish holistic health centers. With financial support from the Kellogg Foundation, several centers were created. Although the centers demonstrated abilities to provide holistic care, they were too costly to sustain and eventually closed (Paul, 2000). One lesson learned from the holistic health canters was that the nurses were the unifying link between the faith-based community and medical community. In 1984, Westberg persuaded officials from Lutheran General Hospital to partner with six faith-based communities to establish a parish nurse program (Westberg, 1987). This first parish nurse model extended even the biopsychosocial models of care by including a spiritual dimension as a component important to human health.

PARISH NURSE MODELS

By 1992, more than 1,500 parish nurses served in many types of places of worship (Hilton, 1993; King, Lakin, & Striepe, 1993). Although parish nurse programs began in Christian churches (e.g., Protestant and Roman Catholic), the programs grew to include various other religious faiths. Christians and Jews share values such as "reverence for life, concern for human welfare, wholeness, and the Hebrew Bible" (Chase–Ziolet & Holst, 1999, p. 200), bringing parish nurses to Jewish settings. Although perspectives vary among faith-based organizations, one value of parish nurse programs is that churches, synagogues, and other places of worship are already established as powerful influences in the spiritual and emotional lives of members (Westberg, 1987). They offer nurses an opportunity to expand the spiritual and emotional influences to encompass a physical health dimension. The growth of parish nurse programs is a result of various collaborative partnerships with faith-based organizations.

Health Services Parish Nursing

Some parish nurses work under Health Services Parish Nurse programs, a collaborative effort between area hospitals and churches (Djupe & Solari-Twadell, 1995). According to Westberg's (1999) institutional-based model, the nurse is employed by the hospital and receives salary and benefits. After a phase-in period, some churches assume the nurse's salary. The hospital's board appoints a committee, including a physician and chaplain, to supervise the nurse. The nurse receives up to 6 hr of training twice a month at a local hospital and ministers to her assigned faith-based organization. The key to a successful program is matching the right nurse with the right congregation (Boario, 1993).

Volunteer Model

A second approach to parish nurse programs relies on volunteers. Church officials apply to area hospitals to partner in a volunteer model of parish nursing. In most cases, the nurse is a member of the church; however, if no volunteer comes forth, the hospital assists the church in selecting a nurse. The nurse receives informational and instrumental support from hospital staff, including assistance with wellness program planning and relevant health information from professionals. Generally, the church's Outreach Ministry Council supervises the nurse.

Nurse Parishioner Model

A third approach to parish nursing programs falls outside the rubric of a formal alliance. Some nurses from the congregation volunteer to assume the role of parish nurse and act as "catalysts for holistic health and for enhancing caring" (Striepe & King, 1993, p. 13). Others volunteer to act in more informal ways to involve church members with activities designed to promote health. For example, they might lead an exercise class or teach nutrition classes. These nurses rely on each other and health ministry committee members for insight and guidance.

In sum, parish nurses are expected to be educators, counselors, support group organizers, community liaisons, role models, and promoters of health (Hilton, 1993; Solari-Twadell, 1999). They establish referrals for professional services, fulfill community service demands, and garner volunteers to augment routine services (Solari-Twadell &Westberg, 1991) but do not generally engage in hands-on nursing, practice medicine, or duplicate services available through community agencies. A parish nurse represents the community and is a "believer ... in God, clients, nursing, herself, and in a better world" (Solari-Twadell, 1999, p. 24). Hilton (1993) posited that what parish nurses may do best is communicate with faith members in a unique relationship tied to the blending of physical, emotional, and spiritual wellness.

Historically, parish nurse programs have been investigated from a technical skills perspective, emphasizing the need for nurses to have knowledge of community health services and skills to assess community client needs (Solari-Twadell, 1999). This formative investigation considers the following question to address the relationship-building side of parish nursing:

RQ: How do parish nurses view their role and the benefits from partnering with faith-based organizations to meet faith members' physical, emotional, and spiritual wellness?

METHOD

Participants and Procedures

Parish nurses ($N = 25$) were interviewed in person ($n = 14$) or by telephone ($n = 11$) by Carolyn M. Anderson or volunteer students (senior level and graduate) from a health communication course. All student interviewers had completed at least one basic research class. The participant nurses (all women) ranged in age from 32 to 67 ($M = 51.30$) and all reported completing college degrees. They partnered with the following: Protestant (6), Roman Catholic (3), Lutheran (3), Baptist (3), Presbyterian (1), Episcopalian (2), Methodist (1), nondenominational (2), Unitarian (2), and Church of God (2). Faith communities ranged in size from 100 families to over 8,000 members. Health ministry committees consisted of 3 to 30 members, with most committees ($n = 20$) including clergy, in addition to social workers, physicians, and lay persons.

The interviewers ($n = 20$) received extensive training that included an introduction to and practice in following the interview schedule. Some of the interview statements and questions used in this study were as follows: (a) Describe the health ministry in your faith community, (b) describe your role as a parish nurse, (c) in what ways do you think you help faith members lead healthier lives? emotional lives? spiritual lives? and (d) what are the benefits from partnering with faith-based organizations in meeting faith members' needs for physical, emotional, and spiritual wellness?

The interviews lasted 30 to 40 min. Interviewers took handwritten notes, which were used in data analysis. Open coding, an iterative process whereby data are compared for similarity and difference, was employed (Strauss & Corbin, 1990). Open coding allows for the addition, combination, and revision of content categories, promoting a parsimonious description of the data. First, the author coded the data. Then, two coders worked independently to assess the author's work. The percentage of agreement between the three coders was high (98%), with differences resolved through discussion. A comparison of phone and face-to-face data revealed no major differences and, thus, appeared to contribute minimally to results.

RESULTS

The research question broadly considered how parish nurses view their role and the benefits of partnering with faith-based organizations to meet faith members' physical, emotional, and spiritual wellness. The nurses described their programs as part of formal committees with the goal of promoting health and wellness. Responses included reference to promotion strategies within the faith-based organization such as newsletters and educational clinics. Newsletters were described as valuable sources of health information for faith members as were educational clinics, where faith members come for health screenings (e.g., diabetes and blood pressure). The educational clinics served a much broader function, however, as they provided a setting for dialogue with faith members about a broad array of health and wellness issues and relationship-building, leading to the provision of social support, a primary theme associated with the data that revealed itself in two distinct ways.

Holistic Approach to Support: Care Without Walls

The overwhelming consistency in participant responses revealed an emphasis on providing social support. The examples illustrated that a holistic approach to such support included both an emphasis on faith practices and a willingness to extend support and care beyond the walls of faith-based organizations. Excerpts from educational clinic experiences reveal how the faith-based organizational setting provided opportunities for parish nurses to build trust, often through provision of emotional support, as illustrated in the following participant's excerpt:

> An older man in the community was scared about losing his friend who was dying. He came to the blood pressure screening and began to talk about his fears. I was able to help him work through his feelings.

Another participant exemplifies the provision of emotional support given beyond church walls:

> A parishioner was dying of cancer at home. She was concerned that she was a burden and not able to give anymore. I was able to help her see that just her upbeat attitude was a gift to others and her strong faith was a huge gift to others battling cancer.

In the former example, the church-based blood pressure screening afforded a space for talking about and seeking emotional support. In the latter case, home visitation granted an opportunity for the nurse to give emotional and esteem support, embracing the parishioner's identity needs.

Parish nurses also recounted many examples of providing tangible support. As noted by one

> At the screening, I was able to determine a problem with hypertension. The faith member had run out of medication and did not have the money to refill the prescription. I was able to help him get it.

Such support again extended beyond the worship sites, continuing to enrich the meaning of holistic care provided by the nurses. Another observed the following:

> A diabetic faith member was not attending church and was on the homebound list. I visited her home and checked the infected toe that was causing her pain and discomfort and recommended a specialist for her to see.

Not surprisingly, the parish nurses often revealed the importance of informational and instrumental support given through worship site health clinics as well. One participant said

> I taught one of my congregate members about their medications and how to take them along with the importance of a correct diet in conjunction with the medications.

Another nurse's recollection revealed the extension of such support beyond worship site settings:

> I showed a woman who was not able to get out of her house a videotape on bladder health. The lady had a bladder problem and was very touched by my making the effort to help educate her.

And still another recalled the following:

> A man had a ruptured aortic aneurysm. His wife found him on the floor and called me to ask what to do. I informed her that I would call 911, come over to the house immediately, and for her not to touch him or roll him over.

In sum, faith members telephoned parish nurses at home for support, health advice, or emergencies. The nurses said that such accessibility was necessary because they were part of the faith community, lived in the neighborhood, and had trusting relationships with members. This suggests a different dimension to holistic care than has been emphasized in prior research. Although worship sites for health promotion activities have been touted as a strategy to increase access to health information and care, the accessibility of parish nurses makes evident that access has dimensions associated with availability beyond worship sites. In turn, this may be related to parishioners' comfort levels in seeking both information and care from parish nurses.

Parish Nurse Identity: Educators and Motivators

A second major theme associated with social support was revealed in these interviews, addressing the parish nurse's identity. Prominent in the descriptions associated with parish nurse programs was the nurses' identification with their role. One nurse stated the following:

> We provide a support system for members of the church.

More than that, however, parish nurses talked about their role in providing motivational support:

> [We] provide the initiative to take care of themselves. Teach them better health. Our ministry helps parishioners become more educated, which in turn helps them lead healthier lives.

Although parish nurses' identity statements convey a generosity of spirit that contributes to their community-based activities, the foundation for that is clearly drawn from an inner source, illustrated in statements such as the following:

> The parishioners live healthier lives because they learn to live more spiritual lives.

Another illustration exemplifying the inward focus follows:

The role of prayer in illness and disease control are the same. It heals the person spiritually and mentally prepares them for what is going to happen.

Still another nurse noted the following:

In a religious setting such as ours people can learn to see health issues as a natural part of the cycle of life. It helps to normalize the experience of "being a patient" when the patient can see their sickness in a religious framework.

Even more directly, one nurse stated that

There is a connection between your mind, body, and spirit. Prayer is the way to access this connection.

Another said the following:

People who pray and have a strong faith cope better, and have less stress thus promoting an overall sense of well being.

In sum, the parish nurses interviewed for this project affirm the value of these programs in providing a model of community-based health care that makes use of faith-based organizations for the delivery of health information, promotion, and care. The participants' experiences enrich the meaning of holistic care, relating it not only to support for emotional, physical, and spiritual well-being but accessibility beyond the walls of worship sites, as nurses attain parishioners' trust.

DISCUSSION

Providing a formative look into parish nursing from the perspective of building relationships between nurses and parishioners revealed important insights about the success of these programs beyond identifying how they organize to deliver care through places of worship. Results indicate that the formal organizational strategies used by faith-based organizations to communicate about health issues to faith members led to important opportunities for parish nurses to minister directly to the physical, interpersonal, and spiritual needs of faith members, sometimes extending outside worship sites. Parish nurses provided support beyond what is typically available in traditional models of health care delivery, bridging the worlds of medicine and religion to link with people (Grace, 1999). Specifically, parish nurses prayed with faith members, found resources for them, spent time with them, were accessible to them, and played a strong, nurturing role for faith members. These types of social support were motivated by intrinsic values associated with the role of spirituality as critical to promoting holistic health. Traditional models of health strive to address the physical concerns of patients, but alternative models that attempt to define health and well-being as multidimensional constructs should encompass spirituality and social support. These factors may be pivotal in understanding health communication between caregivers and patients as well as health-related outcomes.

Ethical Concerns

Parish nurse programs are examples of community-based efforts to deliver health care through existing faith-based organizations. Faith-based endeavors may be supported by government agencies as a strategy to address many health-related issues deemed politically and socially salient, resulting in opportunities for faith-based organizations to sponsor parish nursing programs. Although the utilization of faith-based communities may be an excellent strategy to deliver services, faith-based efforts should not eclipse the delivery of health care through other sources and they also should not be a substitute for efforts to increase access in rural and other underserved areas (Griffin, 1999). Moreover, care should be taken to insure parishioners' confidentiality, with extra efforts taken when parish nurses serve small faith communities where informal information networks flourish. Additionally, some faith-based organizations ask members to disclose sins and seek forgiveness in a private confession or publicly in front of faith members. This has implications for self-disclosure for both faith members and parish nurses such that the boundaries of care may be less clear within faith-based health ministries. For example, if drinking alcohol is considered a "sin" and a parish nurse is treating a faith member for problems associated with alcoholism—where does the role of the parish nurse end? Should she add this person to prayer lists, talk with the patient about the "sinfulness" of the addiction, or simply provide immediate care and individual spiritual support through prayer and conversation? Thus, the ethical boundaries of the role of health ministers may be blurred at times.

Limitations and Future Research

Although participants in this project represent a broad range of Christian denominations and size of worship populations, they do not represent the full range of parish nurse programs or participants. Also, not all parish nurses are comfortable with aspects of their role, such as praying with another (Schnorr, 1999). This study did not capture the involvement of parish nurses with such reservations and thus, lacks insights into how such reticence contributes to individual identities associated with being a parish nurse. Attention to this type of issue by researchers is important because parish nurses are expected to pray with faith members and serve as role models in prayer (Striepe & King, 1993). Insights about varied nursing communicator styles to involve parishioners, strategies for persuading faith members to engage in healthier behaviors, and strategies to protect faith members' confidentiality are but a few areas where communication theory may be fruitfully applied to extend these findings. This research is one formative step toward understanding the roles of health care delivery systems interacting with faith-based organizations.

REFERENCES

Bille, D. A. (1981). The approach to health care in three American minorities. In D. A. Bille (Ed.), *Practical approaches to patient teaching* (pp. 85–94). Boston: Little, Brown.

Boario, M. T. (1993). Mercy model: Church-based healthcare in the inner city. *Journal of Christian Nursing, 10,* 20–33.

Carson, V. B. (1989). *Spiritual dimensions of nursing practice.* Philadelphia: Saunders.

Chase-Ziolet, M., & Holst, L. E. (1999). Parish nursing in diverse traditions. In P. A. Solari-Twadell & M. A. McDermott (Eds.), *Parish nursing: Promoting whole person health within faith communities* (pp. 195–204). Thousand Oaks, CA: Sage.

Djupe, A. M., & Solari-Twadell, A. (1995).The parish nurse. *Home Health Focus, 2,* 53.

du Pre, A. (2000). *Communicating about health: Current issues and perspectives.* Mountain View, CA: Mayfield.

Engle, G. L. (1977). The need for a new medical model: A challenge for biomedicine. *Science, 196,* 129–136.

Grace, H. K. (1999). Foreword. In P. A. Solari-Twadell & M. A. McDermott (Eds.), *Parish nursing: Promoting whole person health within faith communities* (pp. xv–xvii). Thousand Oaks, CA: Sage.

Griffin, J. (1999). Parish nursing in rural communities. In P. A. Solari-Twadell & M. A. McDermott (Eds.), *Parish nursing: Promoting whole person health within faith communities* (pp. 75–82). Thousand Oaks, CA: Sage.

Health Ministries Association, Inc. (2001). *People of faith working together for healthier communities.* Atlanta, GA: Author.

Hilton, D. (1993). *New horizons for the church's involvement in health: The church as a healing community.* Brunswick, GA: MAP International.

King, J. M., Lakin, J. A., & Striepe, N. (1993). Coalition building between public health nurses and parish nurses. *Journal of Nursing Administration, 23*(2), 27–31.

Kirschner, G. (1999). Parish nurse and physician relationship in serving the congregation. In P. Solari-Twadell & M. A. McDermott (Eds.), *Parish nursing: Promoting whole person health within faith communities* (pp. 145–150). Thousand Oaks, CA: Sage.

Lawrence, R. J., (2002). The witches' brew of spirituality and medicine. *The Society of Behavioral Medicine, 24,* 74–76.

Ludwig-Beymer, P., & Sarran, H. S. (1999). Parish nurse–physician partnerships: A continuum of care. In P. A. Solari-Twadell & M. A. McDermott (Eds.), *Parish nursing: Promoting whole person health within faith communities* (pp. 151–160). Thousand Oaks, CA: Sage.

Paul, P. (2000). The history of the relationship between nursing and faith traditions. In M. B. Clark & J. K. Olson (Eds.), *Nursing within a faith community: Promoting health in times of transition* (pp. 59–73). Thousand Oaks, CA: Sage.

Schnorr, M. (1999). Spiritual caregiving: A key component of parish nursing. In P. A. Solari-Twadell & M. A. McDermott (Eds.), *Parish nursing: Promoting whole person health within faith communities* (pp. 43–54). Thousand Oaks, CA: Sage.

Sloan, R. P., & Bagiella, E. (2002). Claims about religious involvement and health outcomes. *The Annals of Behavioral Medicine, 24,* 14–21.

Solari-Twadell, P. A. (1999). The emerging practice of parish nursing. In P. A. Solari-Twadell & M. A. McDermott (Eds.), *Parish nursing: Promoting whole person health within faith communities* (pp. 3–24). Thousand Oaks, CA: Sage.

Solari-Twadell, P. A., & Westberg, G. (1991). Body, mind, and soul. *Health Progress, 72,* 24–28.

Strauss, A. L., & Corbin, J. M. (1990). *Basics of qualitative research: Grounded theory procedures and techniques.* Thousand Oaks, CA: Sage.

Striepe, J. M., & King, J. M. (1993). Basics for beginning a parish nurse program. *Journal of Christian Nursing, 10,* 10–15.

Westberg, G. (1987). *The parish nurse.* Park Ridge, IL: National Parish Nurse Resource Center.

Westberg, G. (1999). A personal historical perspective of whole person health and the congregation. In P. A. Solari-Twadell & M. A. McDermott (Eds.), *Parish nursing: Promoting whole person health within faith communities* (pp. 35–42). Thousand Oaks, CA: Sage.

Wylie, L. J. (1990). The mission of health and the congregation. In P. A. Solari-Twadell, A. M. Djupe, & M. A. McDermott (Eds.), *Parish nursing: The developing practice* (pp. 11–26). Park Ridge, IL: International Parish Nurse Resource Center.

HEALTH COMMUNICATION, *16*(1), 129–130

The Church's Role in
Health and Wholeness

Michael Long
Senior Minister
Roswell United Methodist Church

Christians believe that in Jesus's life on earth, he was known as a great teacher, a charismatic leader, and a compassionate healer. Some scholars believe that Jesus spent at least one third of his time in healing ministries. The Old Testament, especially the book of Leviticus, offers common sense guidelines that helped to prevent the spread of illness and disease. The Psalms speak of healing and wholeness made possible through a relationship with a loving Lord. The Judeo–Christian tradition recognizes the importance of health, wholeness, and healing. A relationship based on faith in a caring God can provide health in all its fullness. Gary Gunderson (1997) stated the following: "Faith needs the language of health to understand how it applies to life, health needs the language of faith in order to find its larger context, its meaning" (p. 4).

To be whole persons, we realize that health integrates our spiritual, physical, intellectual, emotional, and social lives. Therefore, health can be experienced in relationships with God and others; health involves a willingness to change; and health is a choice. Local congregations can become centers of healing, caring, and teaching. Through regular healing services, prayers offered for those in hospitals, and various grief and support groups, people experience the church as a place of healing. Some churches provide Stephen Ministers who offer caring ministry by walking with someone during a time of pain or difficulty; other churches have care groups who "check up" on each other and offer caring assistance as needed. Many churches also provide teaching opportunities concerning health and wholeness issues. More and more churches offer a Parish Nurse ministry. The Parish Nurse in our church speaks to various groups about wellness issues, offers periodic screenings of all kinds, provides annual flu shots, conducts health fairs, and oversees quarterly blood drives.

Requests for reprints should be sent to Michael Long, Doctor of Ministry, Senior Minister, Roswell United Methodist Church, 814 Mimosa Blvd., Roswell, GA 30075.

Many doctors and nurses believe in the power of prayer. Even in these days of separation between church and state issues, doctors are rediscovering the power of prayer in a patient's healing; some medical schools even include classes on how to talk with patients about their faith. The churches are not mandating doctors to pray with their patients; however, from the doctor's personal faith experience and from the patients' desire for prayer, flows the healing comfort and power of a healer's prayer for his or her patient. Many studies indicate that prayer makes a difference in a person's recovery.

Since the beginning of recorded history, the Bible has addressed the importance of wholeness. Jesus provided compassionate healing that met physical, emotional, social, and spiritual needs. The faith community has always valued the importance of health and caring; therefore, communities experience hospitals, medical centers, nursing homes, rehabilitation centers, and counseling centers sponsored and supported by churches who believe in healing. Into the 21st century, the church continues to promote health and caring as it encourages all of God's children to experience the wholeness of life.

REFERENCE

Gunderson, G. (1997). *Deeply woven roots.* Minneapolis, MN: Augsburg Fortress.